# THE CONTROLLED CLINICAL TRIAL

## *An Analysis*

Harris L. Coulter, Ph.D.

CENTER FOR EMPIRICAL MEDICINE

PROJECT CURE

Washington, D.C.
1991

The author wishes to thank the following for permission to quote from the sources listed:

Blackwell Scientific Publications Ltd., for permission to quote from *Clinical Trials*, F. Neil and Susan Johnson, editors. Copyright, 1977, Blackwell Scientific Publications.

William & Wilkins Co., Baltimore, for permission to quote from *Clinical Judgment*, by Alvan Feinstein. Copyright, 1967, Williams & Wilkins Co.

*The Controlled Clinical Trial: An Analysis*

Publishers' addresses:

**Center for Empirical Medicine**
4221 45th Street, NW
Washington, DC 20016

**Project Cure**
1101 Connecticut Avenue, NW
Suite 403
Washington, DC 20036


Coulter, Harris L. (Harris Livermore), 1932-
    The controlled clinical trial : an analysis / Harris L. Coulter.
    165 p. 2.5 cm.
    Includes bibliographical references.
    ISBN 0-916386-04-X: $12.00
    1. Drugs — Testing. 2. Clinical trials. I. Title.
    [DNLM: 1. Clinical Trials. QV 771 C8548c]
RM301.27.C68 1991
615.5'8'0287 — dc20
DNLM/DLC                                                      91-8016
for Library of Congress                                      CIP

# CONTENTS

# INTRODUCTION

Prior to 1962 the normal procedure, in use a century or longer, for bringing a new medicine to professional attention was to elicit testimonials from a handful of physicians. These were then employed in the manufacturer's marketing campaign. (1)

While this horse-and-buggy technique readily lent itself to abuse, before 1945 it was little criticized. The pharmaceutical industry had a low rate of innovation, and new entities were introduced into commerce in a way which satisfied all parties.

But the drug industry was transformed by World War II. The rate of innovation accelerated, and medicines such as penicillin and the other antibiotics seemed amazingly effective. The postwar marketplace rapidly became saturated with new entities and combinations, the period 1954-1959, especially, being marked by "fantastic growth." (2)

In 1939 Americans consumed a total of 182,000,000 drug prescriptions, four out of five being compounded on the premises by the druggist. By 1958 the volume had mounted to 655,000,000, and nine tenths were ready-made by the manufacturer. (3)

Gross sales worldwide of U.S prescription drug products increased from $1.43 billion in 1950 to $2.86 billion in 1960 to $6.853 billion in 1970 to $21.9 billion in 1980 to $51.5 billion in 1989. The number of new entities rose from less than 10 in 1940 to 45 in 1949, to 50 in 1953, and to a peak of 60 in 1959. (4)

Furthermore, each new entity was accompanied by five or six drug combinations, the total number of new combinations introduced on the market reaching a high-water mark of 280 in 1955. (5)

This increased volume of production demanded a technique for separating more effective medicines from less effective. The answer was the "controlled clinical trial" (CCT) or "randomized clinical trial" (RCT), first suggested in the 1930s by the British statistician, Austin Bradford Hill.

The results, of course, like physicians' testimonials, could then be usefully employed in manufacturers' publicity campaigns.

While some controlled clinical research had been performed in Great Britain and the United States before the war, the first major controlled clinical trial of a new drug was the 1946-1948 British study of streptomycin in tuberculosis, for which Hill provided statistical support.* (6)

The use of the controlled trial spread slowly in the 1950s as manufacturers realized its value in their unceasing maneuvering for market position and market share. Hedley Atkins, President of the Royal College of Surgeons, told Austin Hill at this time that his contribution to medicine "was as important and valuable as the discovery of penicillin." (7)

The real impetus for their proliferation came with the 1962 adoption of the Kefauver-Harris Amendments to the United States Food, Drug, and Cosmetic Act. Prior to this time manufacturers had been required only to furnish evidence of "safety," but the 1960-1961 tragedy of thalidomide, when 10,000 women in Europe, Asia, and the United States gave birth to deformed babies through taking an apparently innocent sleeping pill during pregnancy, led to a strengthening of the American drug law.** Henceforth "substantial evidence" of efficacy became a requirement.

---

*Emblematic of the later history of the clinical trial is the fact that the streptomycin study, extolled then and since as a breakthrough in medicine, in fact yielded disappointing results: the treated cases showed improvement only for three months and thereafter began to deteriorate. (Medical Research Council, 782)

The new law defined "substantial evidence" rather vaguely as "adequate and well-controlled investigations, including clinical investigations" — words which lent themselves to various interpretations. A 1983 *Background Paper* on clinical trials produced by the U.S. Congress's Office of Technology Assessment (OTA) noted:

> The authors of the 1962 amendments were not necessarily thinking of RCTs when they wrote the phrase "adequate and controlled studies." That language may simply have been obtained from testimony in hearings. The phrase was used as the scientific analog of the legal phrase "substantial evidence" (i.e., more than an iota, less than a preponderance). (8)

In due course, however, the language of the law was interpreted by the U.S. Food and Drug Administration (FDA) to mean "randomized" and "controlled" clinical trials.

Since 1962 most new drugs in the United States have been tested for "efficacy" by the clinical trial. A minimum of two controlled studies, preferably randomized, is usually required for each indication. (9) From 5000 to 10,000 clinical trials are conducted every year throughout the world, with several hundred thousand patients participating.

In the United States about 7000 physicians are engaged in clinical trials, with 2000 or so being active in any given year. (10) Since manufacturers do not like to discuss the development of new products, information on clinical trials is not routinely divulged, and the very existence of an ongoing clinical trial constitutes a "trade secret." (11)

Although the public believes the clinical trial to be a model of scientific method, the profession's attitude is more

---

**Since thalidomide turned out to be highly unsafe, its sale in the United States was already barred by the pre-1962 Food and Drug Law. It was, in fact, an "effective" tranquilizer. While this drug was never marketed commercially in the United States, it was used here on an experimental basis, leading to the birth of about twenty deformed babies. For a clinical trial of thalidomide see L. Lasagna, 1960.

tempered. A 1987 consensus conference in Lugano, Switzerland, representing several hundred specialists in CCT methodology responded as follows when asked why these trials are in a state of "crisis":

- they are corrupted by too many purely commercial trials (74% agreed with this statement)
- trial protocols are often inadequate (72%)
- their results are often ambiguous and uninterpretable (58%)
- they are too expensive (50%)
- they have low priority as a research activity (41%)
- public pressure prevents many physicians from participating in them (35%)
- the gap between the CCT and clinical reality cannot be bridged (33%)
- they violate the doctor-patient relationship (30%)(12)

The *British Medical Journal* editorialized on the Lugano meeting as follows:

> If there is a crisis, it probably stems from doctors' reluctance to accept their uncertainty about much of what they practice. The randomized trial is still misunderstood and underused and is certainly not accepted as an integral part of a professional practice that should constantly strive to improve the safety and efficacy of its treatments. (M.B.Bracken, M.D., 1987)(13)

In the following pages we will examine these and other issues to reach an understanding of the present status and the prospects for the "controlled clinical trial."

# I. HUMAN VARIETY IN HEALTH AND DISEASE

The intractable problem which the clinical trial is supposed to resolve is that of human variety.

A Greek physician wrote in the second century A.D.:

> The number of diseases and their accompanying symptoms are endless, owing to the isolation of each case ... We understand by endlessness the variations in their degrees and arrangement which complicate the diseases and their symptoms through some of them preceding and some following others.
>
> In the almost endless variety of their diseases and the symptoms of them, the sick themselves differ from one another ... What is more manifold, more complicated, and more varied than disease? How does one discover that a disease is the same as another disease in all its characteristics? Is it by the number of symptoms or by their strength and power? For if a thing be itself, then in my opinion, it must be itself in all these characteristics, for if even one of them is lacking, it is perverted, and it ceases to be itself. (1)

This lament has been repeated by physicians of every subsequent generation: how is reliable medical knowledge to be developed when the patients themselves manifest such a dazzling variety? How is the physician to find solid ground in this heterogeneity?

5

The variety of disease is rooted in the physiological multiformity manifested by any group of "normal," "healthy," old or young, men and women.

The physiologist Roger Williams, of the University of Texas, has devoted particular attention to the dimensions of biological variation in health. In several writings he has shown that supposedly "normal" young men manifest very different metabolic patterns; these differences, he states, "may be quite large and of more than academic interest."

> While healthy young men of the same height and weight may resemble one another in their overall oxygen consumption, specific chemical reactions may take place, under basal conditions, five or ten times as fast in one individual as in another. Perhaps the most direct extensive evidence on this point is based upon differences in enzyme levels and enzyme efficiencies. Perhaps next to this in importance is the fact that there are wide individual differences among "normals" with respect to several endocrine activities, and there is also anatomical evidence of substantial differences in endocrine patterns ... The overall conclusion seems clear that, while the body chemistry of each individual is subject to some change with environmental conditions, each individual would, if subjected to the same stress and given the same food, exhibit a highly distinctive metabolic pattern. This pattern is genetically determined and undoubtedly correlated with his distinctive set of organ weights and activities. (2)

Williams goes on to claim, for instance, that probably less than 3% of persons in "normal" health need to consume the "minimum daily requirements" or "recommended dietary allowances" (of vitamins and minerals) so beloved of the government's standard-setting agencies. As he puts it, there is no "normal" requirement for the five major vitamins and minerals (calcium, iron, lysine, thiamine, and riboflavin). The typical healthy individual has a "normal" requirement for one or two of these and thoroughly "abnormal" requirements (i.e., much higher or lower) for the remainder.

"Normal" individuals yield not only average, or nearly average, values, but also values which may be distinctly high or low, or highly variable. In our experience with control young men we have never found one who exhibited a pattern which was free from distinctive variations from the average. (3)

This sort of conclusion should not be startling. If every individual has a different set of fingerprints, why should everyone have the same riboflavin requirement?

Humans differ in this respect from animals, especially laboratory animals. Inbred, and even "outbred," strains of rats and guinea-pigs are far more uniform than humans. This complicates any effort to predict the reaction of humans to a given pharmacologic substance merely from the results of animal studies. (4)

Human metabolism changes with age. The liver of the fetus, for instance, contains large quantities of iron and copper, while after birth both levels decline; then, after the first year of life the iron content starts to rise, while that of copper remains low. (5)

The proportions of different cell types and rates of cell division continually change during growth and development, suggesting equally substantial changes in metabolic activity. After age thirty, for example, there is a decline in the number of fibers in the nervous system, in nerve conduction, basal metabolism, cardiac output, and pulmonary function, while the rate of cell turnover in the skin and gums increases.

Sexual differences are significant for metabolism. Men and women have different blood composition, women's blood being characterized by less hemoglobin and red cells and less plasma protein. In most species of animals the organs reveal sex-related differences in metabolic capacity and response.

Diet has a profound effect on metabolism; this holds true especially for protein intake, since it affects albumin production by the liver. In the adult, albumin comprises 60% of the protein in the plasma and extracellular fluid; in the child this can be as high as 75%. About 14 grams of albumin are manufactured every day by the liver of the "average 70-

kilogram man" who is the chief subject of research in physiology. An equivalent amount is destroyed every day as well. Hence the protein content of the diet affects all of the body's physiologic processes.

The human body contains about 200,000 different types of protein, each of which, in function of the individual's genetic material (DNA, chromosomes), is subject to a degree of variation.

The metabolism undergoes variation from season to season and from day to night. Body temperature is lowest upon awakening, while plasma steroid and iron levels in the blood are highest at that time. Thereafter the temperature rises, while plasma steroid and iron levels decline. Body temperature is different in the tropics and also in arctic zones; in women it varies with the menstrual cycle. (6)

The metabolism is greatly affected by emotional stress, which acts through the pituitary gland on the production of adrenal steroids. And these steroids, in turn, affect the body's enzyme activity, immunologic defenses, and other major processes.

All of these factors stamp a degree of uniqueness on every individual.

But the ultimate uniqueness is conferred by variations in a group of proteins found in the blood known as "immune globulins."

They come in five classes, the largest being gamma-globulin (IgG). Each globulin class is comprised of four peptide chains, two "light" and two "heavy," which make up the basic structure of the molecule. In the human population a total of 23 inheritable variations in portions of basic chains of IgG have been identified—20 in the heavy chains and three in the light chains. So, merely in this one subcategory of protein, gamma globulin, overall variety is determined by the  permutations and combinations of 23 inheritable features.

Specific changes in immune globulins represent reactions to alien substances (usually proteins) known as "antigens." When introduced into the body, "antigen" acts in ways not yet understood to alter the makeup of immune globulin —

known as "antibody formation." "Antibody" then combines with the alien antigen and removes it from the host organism. This reactivity of the immune globulins is — again in an unknown way — stamped upon them so that, when exposed a second time to the same antigen, they can respond more rapidly to combine with it and remove it from the body.

Even the reaction of the same individual to the same antigen can vary with circumstances. Elvin Kabat, who in 1948 discovered the A, B, and O blood groupings, wrote in 1976:

> If human serum albumin is injected into a group of rabbits to stimulate the formation of antibodies, each rabbit may produce antibody to any or all of the antigenic determinants on the albumin molecule. The proportion of antibody to any determinant of the total may vary from rabbit to rabbit and may change even in a single rabbit as the injections of antigens are continued; occasional animals may fail to form antibody to one or more determinants ... We speak of this as one of the several manifestations of the heterogeneity of antibodies. The extraordinary magnitude of this heterogeneity is the unique characteristic of antibodies (and of immunoglobulins) ... (7)

The striking variety of possible immunologic responses to antigens has been, and remains, a puzzle to biologists and physicians. How many different antibodies can the human organism generate? One textbook of immunology states: "Estimates (perhaps better described as guesses) of this number have ranged from a lower limit of 100,000 to 'effectively infinite.'" (8)

And, as noted, the record of the individual's reaction to these antigens is stamped upon the immune globulins and becomes an intrinsic part of his makeup. Rene Dubos, one of the world's leading bacteriologists and medical philosophers, wrote in his classic *Reason Awake* (1970):

> It is certain that the phrase, "human constitution," implies much more than the genetic endowment. The

characteristics of a person and the responses (healthy or pathological) he makes to the environment are profoundly conditioned by the past experiences he has embodied in his biological and moral being. (9)

Thus, the individual's *history* becomes part of his uniqueness.

Investigations of the human organism find diversity and heterogeneity wherever they are sought.

This includes varying responses to medication.

When U.S. troops during the Korean War were administered a quinine-derived antimalarial pill, black soldiers were found, in many cases, to become anemic, and the cause was seen to lie in a deficiency of a particular red-cell enzyme which affects about 10% of American blacks. This deficiency altered their reaction to sulfa compounds, headache medicines containing phenacetin, and some medicines used to treat kidney and bladder infections. (10)

Blacks, Caucasians, and Chinese are known to respond differently to alcohol, cocaine, ephedrine, morphine, and many other medications. (11)

The antidiarrheal drug *Enterobioform* which is entirely harmless to Caucasians has been implicated as a cause of eye, nerve, and brain damage in more than 10,000 Japanese. (12)

Women with blood-type A are three times more likely to develop thrombophlebitis from birth-control pills than women of blood types B or O. (13)

Some individuals can acquire a lethally high fever from the commonly used anesthetic, halothane. Drugs such as sulfadimidine or isoniazid are metabolized at different rates by different individuals and thus have different effects. (14)

The phenomenon of penicillin allergy is also well known. From 15 to 40 of each 10,000 persons administered penicillin develop a severe reaction, while one patient in 5000 dies from such a reaction — for a total of 300 deaths per year. (15)

The intractable problem of "side effects" or "adverse reactions" to drugs itself reflects the varying metabolisms of the patients taking these drugs. No drug affects everyone in the same way; and any drug will affect the metabolism of some recipients in undesired ways. (16) Children are especially unpredictable, sometimes manifesting a stronger reaction, sometimes a weaker one, and sometimes one which is entirely "paradoxical." (17)

The peculiar features of an individual, which set him apart from others and determine the specificity of his reaction, have historically been called his "idiosyncrasy." Roger Williams has suggested that the individual's "idiosyncrasy" is the most important feature of his illness and that a systematic knowledge of such idiosyncrasies would enable physicians to cure illnesses more rapidly and efficiently:

> The character of these distinctive metabolic patterns is directly related to the susceptibility of individuals to many diseases of obscure etiology, as well as to others belonging in the infectious, nutritional, metabolic, malignant, degenerative, geriatric, mental, or other categories... the "seeds" of many of these causes of death and disability probably reside in the "normal" young men at age twenty and may be discoverable at that time if we take the pains to find them. Even those individuals who die in their later years of infectious diseases may exhibit, at age twenty, distinctive signs of susceptibility... the purpose of such an investigation would be to ferret out the "abnormalities" rather than the "normalities" existing in these "normal" young men. (18)

In other words, Williams regards the specific metabolic *peculiarities* of the individual as more significant for present and future health than those areas of the metabolism where each young man overlaps with all the others.

Belief in the likelihood of idiosyncratic and "abnormal" reactions to medicines is a feature of American popular culture. In 1972 the FDA commissioned a study of public opinion on medical matters and found, to its surprise and displeasure, that "millions of consumers appear to be basing health decisions on the idea that, since there are individual differences in people, there is a chance that almost any treatment may be beneficial. They reason that the only way to find out whether something works is to try it." The FDA's reaction to this finding was censorius in the extreme: "a serious oversimplification ... an uncritical trial and error approach ... Rational judgment is ruled out, since no evidence that a practice failed to help other people is sufficient to eliminate the possibility that it may appear to help someone." (19)

The FDA qualified this attitude of the American public as "rampant empiricism."

And, indeed, the opinion of the FDA reflects that of the majority of physicians — who are convinced that, for purposes of medical and pharmacologic research, the individual's "idiosyncrasy" or "abnormality" is less important than the features he possesses in common with others, i.e., his "normalities." Louis Lasagna, M.D., prominent pharmacologist and medical educator, has written (1964) that emphasis on the patient's "idiosyncrasy":

> can, unfortunately, be used in an anti-intellectual sense to suggest that medical treatment is inherently a mystical process, which cannot be quantified, analyzed, or communicated. Perhaps the most frequently cited epitomization of this last interpretation is the "no-patient-is-like-any-other-patient" ploy. We are, to be sure, all different from one another, and it is probably true that one could listen to hundreds of lungs during the pneumonia season and not find two that sounded exactly alike. But this is not the same as saying that there are no common features in such patients or that therapeutically one starts from scratch every time one faces a patient with pneumonia. If this were so, medical teaching would be impossible and the practice of medicine chaos, or at least anarchy. The problem of individual differences is indeed a challenging one ... but it is no reason for paralytic despair. (20)

Whether or not an occasion for "paralytic despair," human variety is the fundamental issue in the "controlled clinical trial." This procedure will be scientifically valid only if it can accommodate, and allow for, the heterogeneity of human sickness. If this heterogeneity is ignored or assumed out of existence, the "controlled clinical trial" must be judged a failure.

## II. THE DISEASE ENTITY

The assumption that patients have "common features" which can be "quantified, analyzed, and communicated," and that treatment should be grounded on these common features, is the theoretical justification for the controlled clinical trial.

The "common features" assumption accepted by Louis Lasagna and most other physicians has never been demonstrated and may be entirely false. But its medical pedigree is no less ancient than the opposed idea of infinite human variety.

The Greeks described tuberculosis, malaria, diarrhoea, dysentery, ophthalmias, and other conditions — all recognized by their typical patterns of signs and symptoms, course, and outcome. In following centuries other "diseases" emerged: leprosy, bubonic plague, cancers, tumors, epilepsy, syphilis, etc.

The seventeenth-century British physician, Thomas Sydenham, distinguished measles from scarlet fever and left accurate pictures of gout, bronchopneumonia, pleuropneumonia, dysentery, chorea, and malaria. Paris physicians in the nineteenth century developed differentiated portraits of tuberculosis, typhus, typhoid, diphtheria, cardiac conditions, and many others.

Today the *International Classification of Diseases* lists 671 categories of "diseases and morbid conditions," each with its subcategories and sub-subcategories. (1)

Every disease name and definition represents professional consensus on the characteristics of this disease process

— i.e., the traits found in all, or nearly all, persons suffering from the given "disease" or "morbid condition." The traits may be taken from pathological anatomy, symptomatology, bacteriology, or biochemistry, but in all cases they are the common features observed in a group of patients suffering from the "same disease."

These disease definitions, these "entities," have played and do play an absolutely central role in the professional life of the doctor. The Danish pathologist, Knud Faber, wrote in 1922:

> The description of a new disease is of extremely great importance in practical medicine. To the physiologist and the worker in the laboratory, morbid categories are subordinate concepts, but to the physician, to the clinician, the reverse is the case; he cannot live, cannot speak, cannot act without them. (2)

The same view has been echoed by more recent writers:

> Not long ago, during the pathology era of medicine, we were concerned mainly with structural changes. With the rise of microbiology the clinical entity shifted to changes based on common etiological factors. More recently we have been concerned with underlying metabolic disturbances. But all of these have simply been devices for tying independent characteristics into a unit of identification ... It is a way of recognizing uniformity among patients and using it as a basis for therapeutic decision. (Theodore Greiner, M.D., 1965)(3)

The physician perceives the "disease," not the patient. He treats the "disease," not the patient.

> Although the primary object of medical science is to improve the health or cure the sickness of the *individual*, the relevant knowledge usually has to be accumulated slowly by the observation of *groups* of individuals ... it is a reversion to primitive ways of think-

ing to say there are no diseases, there are only sick people. (L.J.Witts, M.D. and N.T.J.Bailey, M.D., 1964)(4)

Physicians tend to regard diseases as fixed and permanent natural entities. They accept and use them without a second thought. Ivan Pavlov, the great Russian nineteenth-century physiologist, stated in a 1900 lecture that clinical medicine "in the thousand years of its existence has succeeded in definitely establishing the types of different diseases and in giving a near perfect morphology of the pathological conditions." (5)

But are they right? Was Pavlov right?

Are "diseases" discrete entities which can be readily described and easily distinguished from one another? Is L.J.Witts, M.D., correct when he states:

The semantic and philosophic problems in defining diseases have been exaggerated, for it is no more difficult than defining other biological reactions. (6)

Or is "disease" a continuum, a seamless web of suffering? Are the "diseases" recognized by medicine today nothing more than clusters of symptomatic, biochemical, and pathological data selected by observers as significant for reasons only marginally related to the inherent nature of the patient's morbidity?

The use of ... particular diagnostic terms may lead us to believe that a real disease exists whereas it really indicates our basic ignorance, masked by our ability to make superficial descriptions... As the history of medicine has demonstrated, these shifting similarities which we call entities depend not so much on reality as on the things we are able to measure and choose to see. (Theodore Greiner, M.D., 1965)(7)

The answer to this question is of the utmost importance for our attitude toward the clinical trial. If defining a "disease" is "no more difficult than defining other biological reactions," the testing of medicines against these same "dis-

17

eases" in clinical trials is a straightforward affair. In the opposite case, however, the clinical trial takes on unexpected dimensions of complexity.

Indeed, physicians in recent decades have found the contours of traditional "entities" to be much fuzzier than was suspected by Ivan Pavlov. When closely scrutinized, the entity recedes from view like the Cheshire cat, leaving nothing but an enigmatic smile.

Alvan Feinstein, M.D., professor at the Yale Medical School, has commented extensively on problems of disease definition in his classic *Clinical Judgment* and other writings:

> No other branch of natural science is so imprecise in defining the material exposed to experiment. Although all the diagnoses are made differently, although no uniform standards have been ratified and disseminated, it is commonly believed that rigorous criteria are invariably present. The clinician's capacity for intellectual self-deception is illustrated by the widespread acceptance of this illusion. For most of the "established" diagnoses of modern "disease," standardized criteria do not exist, but are necessary, and must be established for true scientific progress in clinical medicine. For clinicians to improve scientific quality in the treatment of "disease," a basic demand of science is an accurate reproducible identification of "disease." Such identifications will require clinicians to establish and disseminate the specific details of suitable criteria for diagnosis of each "disease" subjected to therapy. (Alvan Feinstein, M.D., 1976)(8)

> The current taxonomy of disease is a polyglot of diverse ideas and names. The available diagnostic terms for disease include different categories of topography, morphology, physiology, biochemistry, microbiology, genetics, "clinical states," syndromes, signs, and habits. (Alvan Feinstein, M.D., 1977)(9)

Probably the major methodological obstacle blocking precise definition of a given disease entity is that symptomatic, pathological, and biochemical data do not necessarily coincide or concur with one another. (10)

Symptoms may not correspond to pathological lesions discovered at autopsy. The patient with duodenal ulcer has no stomach pains. The woman with endometriosis (overgrowth of the mucous lining of the uterus) does not have bleeding and cramps. (11) The man with emphysema has no difficulty breathing. (12) The diabetic does not urinate to excess. (13) The patient with myocardial infarction has no chest pain. (14) William Osler wrote in 1908:

> Extreme sclerosis of the coronary arteries is common, and a large majority of the cases present no symptoms of angina. Even in the case of sudden death due to blocking of an artery, particularly the anterior branch of the coronary artery, there is usually no pain either before or during an attack. (15)

The patient with normal coronary arteries and whose reading on an exercise test is normal, or who has only shortness of breath when walking upstairs, may nonetheless have angina pectoris — described as:

> a disease of unknown evolution, confusing symptomatology, and objective manifestations — such as electrocardiographic abnormalities — which do not correlate well with those symptoms. (O.B.Ross, Jr., M.D., 1967)(16)

Electrocardiograms and angiograms often correlate poorly with other types of cardiac irregularities. (17)

X-ray findings may not correspond to the patient's clinical state: he has a shadow on the lung but no symptoms of tuberculosis. (18)

The same is true for biochemical findings — which may not correlate with either the symptoms or the pathology. The patient has gallstones, but his symptoms are not related to gall-bladder disease. (19) His blood has a high uric acid level, but he has no gout. (20) Nitrogen compounds in the blood of patients with nephritis may be unrelated to tissue changes in the kidneys. (21)

Confusion stems, in part, from the fact that different "diseases" have emerged at different periods of history, and physicians prefer the type of data in vogue at the time of the disease's discovery. But the result may be chaos.

In consequence, textbooks avoid precise symptomatic or pathological definitions of diseases, and physicians must develop their own personal rules of thumb:

> Every clinician has his own criteria for clinical diag-
> nosis of *congestive heart failure, nephrotic syndrome,* and
> *hepatic decompensation,* but no criteria have been stan-
> dardized, and none are used uniformly. Every clini-
> cian has his own criteria for such clinical entities as
> *hypertension* or *coronary artery disease,* but no definitive
> criteria have been established. Every clinical textbook
> contains many remarks about diagnosis of disease,
> but none present the rigorous delineation required of
> scientific criteria... Lacking any formal means of clas-
> sifying clinical observations, the clinician has no place
> to put the information when he communicates with
> himself or with his colleagues ... He cannot speak his
> clinical distinctions well, or think about them clearly,
> or read about them specifically, or write about them
> formally, because he cannot stipulate them — he has
> no ordered taxonomic vocabulary for them. (Alvan
> Feinstein, M.D, 1976)(22)

The categories of "mental illness" are especially problem-atical, since they can rarely be correlated with anatomical or biochemical changes and are established from signs and symptoms alone.

> Mental illnesses resemble many other illnesses also in
> not being understood. Most of them are at present
> classified only by their symptoms. What appears as
> the name of an illness — schizophrenia, hysteria, and
> so forth — stands for an unknown common factor

which is assumed to underlie particular syndromes. Any of these names might disappear overnight if deeper knowledge were to provide a better classification or even to prove that the existing one is without practical value. (Geoffrey Vickers, M.D., 1965)(23)

The current psychiatric debates about systems of classification, the many hypothetical and unconfirmed schemas of "psychodynamic mechanisms," and the concern with etiological inference rather than observational evidence are nosologic activities sometimes reminiscent of those conducted by the medieval taxonomists. (Alvan Feinstein, M.D., 1976)(24)

Though large sums have been poured into psychiatric research, very little is clearly established. Body fluids have been minutely studied for changes in mental illness, but with as little result as if we studied the sewage effluent of a recording studio to establish correlations with the music played ... In psychiatry there are innumerable observations, but virtually no agreed-upon theoretical basis. Systems of classification are changed every few years and vary from country to country. Explanatory theories have no general acceptance and resemble religious systems in that they comfort the believer without being susceptible to proof or disproof. They are subject to fashion and imposed by intrigue. In North America the academic heights have been held mainly by those trained in psychoanalysis, or prepared to pay obeisance to its tenets (often with privately expressed doubts, like those of a priest who has lost his faith). *Credo quia absurdum est* seems to pertain here as in theology. (Elliott Emanuel, M.D., 1978) (25)

"Schizophrenia" is probably the most common mental illness, affecting as many as 30-40% of all mental patients. (26) It has an official definition, characterized as the "core schizophrenia syndrome," consisting of the most commonly encountered symptoms of patients diagnosed as "schizophrenic" in several countries during an International Pilot Study of Schizophrenia. (27)

But few psychiatrists adhere to this definition: "Schizophrenia and essential hypertension are excellent examples of descriptive terms which seem to carry the illusion that concrete disease exists." (28) In one hospital the physicians will call "schizophrenic" only those patients who have been confined two years or more, while others will call these same patients "depressed" or perhaps "brain-damaged," or even "epileptic." (29) The director of the New York State Psychiatric Institute stated in 1979:

> Schizophrenia has been a vast wastebasket. All kinds of psychiatric disorders have been labelled schizophrenic, but I hope that will change. (30)

And while the literature is full of studies of "depression," no precise definition of this condition exists either. (31) A group of patients diagnosed by one physician as "depressed" will contain many whom other diagnosticians would call "schizophrenic," "psychopathic personalities," or even cases of brain damage. (32)

The psychiatrist Thomas Szasz denies the existence of all of these mental illnesses:

> Psychiatrists claim that schizophrenia, depression, alcoholism, smoking, and so on are diseases — but where's the evidence? Every ten years they have different evidence: electrical, chemical, genetic, and so forth. Science is based on honesty, and one thing we know about psychiatrists is that they lie all the time. (33)

Szasz observes that the American Psychiatric Association is always discovering the existence of new mental illnesses — such as "Tobacco Use Disorder" or "Academic Underachievement Disorder." One is reminded of the American antebellum South, where slaves trying to escape North were diagnosed as suffering from "dromomania" (an irrepressible desire to run); or of the recent history of the Soviet Union, where critics of the political order were diagnosed as psychologically maladjusted.

On a few occasions the medical profession has attempted to reach agreed definitions of diseases. In 1956 a committee of the American Rheumatism Association established eleven criteria for the diagnosis of rheumatoid arthritis: the diagnosis is "definite" if the patient manifests five of them, "probable" if three. (34) A committee of the American Heart Association did the same for rheumatic fever in 1963, coming up with five "major" manifestations, three "minor" clinical manifestations, and two "minor" laboratory manifestations. Evidence of preceding streptococcal infection was also required "except in situations in which the rheumatic fever is first discovered after a long latent period from the antecedent infection." The committee concluded that two "major," or one "major" and two "minor" criteria indicated a high probability of the presence of rheumatic fever. (35)

The American Psychiatric Association has adopted a similar approach to the diagnosis of "depression" ("Major Depressive Episode"), listing nine symptoms ("loss of interest in pleasure," "lack of reactivity," "depression regularly worse in the morning," "psychomotor retardation," "significant anorexia or weight loss," etc.) and requiring the patient to manifest at least five of them. (36)

But with this Chinese-restaurant-menu approach two patients can have completely different, or almost completely different, sets of symptoms and laboratory findings and be diagnosed with the "same disease." In rheumatoid arthritis two patients could each have five quite different manifestations, and there would still be one left over. In rheumatic fever two patients could each have two different "major" manifestations (with one left over), or a variety of combinations of "major" and "minor," and still receive the same diagnosis (in "depression" the patient must manifest five out of nine, so there will always be at least a one-symptom overlap between any two "depressed" patients).

However handy such disease definitions may be for medical practice, they do not promote precision in clinical trials.

Another intractable problem arises with the definition of "normal." Disease is defined as a departure from "normality."

For all practical purposes the physician assumes that illness is a deviation from a biologically given norm. (Geoffrey Vickers, M.D., 1965)(37)

Pathological physiology ... is concerned with disturbances in normal physiology. (William A. Sodeman, M.D., 1967)(38)

I believe that disease is fundamentally unnatural ... I believe that disease results generally from biological mistakes. (Lewis Thomas, M.D., 1972) (39)

What exactly does this mean? Roger Williams has shown "normality" to be a fluid concept with no precise boundaries. But if we do not know the limits of the "normal," how can we define departures from it? If we do not know what is "natural," how is the "unnatural" to be recognized?

Patients have been falsely diagnosed as having infectious hepatitis, coronary artery disease, diabetes mellitus, rheumatic carditis, or prostatic carcinoma because of "abnormalities," respectively, in cephalin flocculation, electrocardiographic T-waves, blood sugar, P-R interval, or serum acid phosphatase tests that might have been called "normal" if a better epidemiologic sampling had been used for establishing the basic range of normal. (Alvan Feinstein, M.D, 1976)(40)

Values which are "normal" for one individual (as we have already seen) may be highly "abnormal" for another, indicating severe pathology. So the "wide" and the "narrow" definitions of normality both yield errors. If the definition is "wide," individuals with disease may be diagnosed as "normal"; if it is narrow, the healthy individual may be diagnosed as diseased. (41)

> Because of these deficiencies, there now exist almost no satisfactory absolute criteria for designating a clinical phenomenon as normal or abnormal. (Alvan Feinstein, M.D., 1976)(42)

A dynamic definition of "normality," such as that suggested by W.H.Perkins in 1938, would be much closer to medical reality:

> Health is a state of relative equilibrium of body form and function which results from its successful dynamic adjustment to forces tending to disturb it. *It is not a passive interplay between the body substance and forces impinging upon it, but an an active response of body forces working toward readjustment* ... There is manifested in each of these adjustment phenomena a tendency toward the preservation of a state of limited equilibrium ... As long as the mechanisms involved in physiologic equilibrium are not pressed beyond their powers of restoration within their established limits, and so long as they maintain their ability to dissipate the energies of the factors operating on them to their own levels of tolerance, it may be said that such apparent instability represents the normal. It is impossible to define normal more strictly than this ... [stress added] (43)

But accepting such a definition of "normal health" would require a new set of definitions of disease and a different structure of the clinical trial.

For all these reasons, existing disease names may be, and undoubtedly are, unstable sources of information. Feinstein is of the view, for example, that diagnoses on death certificates are so unreliable as to nullify the comparability of national mortality statistics. (44) The fluidity and friability of these disease definitions, as well as the continuing changes they undergo, also undermine the reliability and comparability of clinical investigations. Those performed today cannot readily be compared with those performed yesterday. Those performed in one country cannot readily be compared with those done in another: for instance, it was discovered in 1964 that U.S. physicians were calling "pulmonary emphysema" what British M.D.s called "chronic bronchitis." (45)

Even those performed at the same time in the same country may employ different diagnostic criteria.

Despite the methodologic difficulties involved in defining the disease entity, no reasonable alternative has been found:

> All these examples of "clinical" diagnoses persist today because the names are necessary. No alternative morphologic, physiologic, or biochemical designations have been adequate to include the wide spectrum of clinical manifestations covered by the "clusters" or to provide a consistent specificity in identifying the affected patients. (Alvan Feinstein, M.D., 1976)(46)

\*   \*   \*   \*   \*   \*   \*

The disease entity is the physician's way of coping with problems of medical practice, specifically, the desire to insert patients into given treatment categories. It does not provide a firm foundation for a structure of scientific medicine. Even though disease names are in steady use, they are merely conveniences for the physician. They correspond to nothing in nature other than vague and shifting similarities among patients.

Two comments may be made.

While these names may be convenient for the physician, they may be less so for the patient — whose particular condition may not quite correspond to the name on his diagnostic chart and whose mode of treatment may not be quite adapted to his true illness. The superficial and careless use of disease names undoubtedly results in much wrongly directed therapy.

And it may be unwise to base the country's whole system for vetting new medicines upon such an inherently unstable concept as the "disease entity."

# III. HOMOGENEITY vs. GENERALIZABILITY

The controlled clinical trial is performed on a "sample" of patients which is divided into a "test" group and a "control" group. The test group receives the new medication (or surgery, or other mode of treatment), while the "controls" receive the previous treatment or perhaps no treatment at all (placebo).

Such a trial rests upon two assumptions of primordial importance: (1) that the sample is "homogeneous," meaning:

> that there are significant similarities among the diseased patients which we can recognize and group into diagnostic categories. If these categories are meaningful, patients presenting the same medical condition will respond to the drug in a similar fashion. (Theodore Greiner, M.D., 1965)(1)

and (2) that the sample is "generalizable," i.e., representative of the larger universe of persons who are or will be suffering from the disease or disease process in question:

> in doing research we often want our conclusions to apply not to the sample alone, but to the original population from which the sample is drawn. The sampling process would usually be undesirable or futile if what we found pertained only to the particular group of people who constituted the sample. We must therefore find a way of getting a sample that

truly represents the population from which it came.
(Alvan Feinstein, M.D., 1977)(2)

These two assumptions have been difficult or impossible
to substantiate. And, in fact, the two desiderata are very much
in conflict with one another.

## Sample Homogeneity

The so-called "homogeneous" group is only the disease
"entity" writ small. The urge to achieve sample "homogeneity" is a rerun of medicine's efforts to define the disease
"entity." Both encounter apparently insurmountable difficulties.

All the traps and snares, all the illusions and pitfalls,
besetting medicine's efforts to define the disease "entity"
affect in equal degree its unwearying search for the "homogeneous" group.

From the very beginning investigators were aware of the
problem of diversity — attributable to "each patient's unique
biological and psychological makeup" — but thought it
unimportant. (3)

> The "controlled experiment" is one of the most im-
> portant concepts in biological experimentation. In
> this there are two or more similar groups (identical
> except for the inherent variability of all biological
> material) ... There will always be variation that de-
> pends on factors not yet understood. It is essential to
> realize the impossibility of obtaining exactly similar
> groups. (W.I.B.Beveridge, M.A., 1957)(4)

However, the results achieved, or not achieved, at length
convinced many authorities that biological heterogeneity
was so great as to jeopardize the outcome of many trials.
Robert Platt, M.D., wrote in 1963:

> In discussions on the ethics of clinical trials there is
> usually a tacit assumption that the trial is scientifically
> sound. This is far from being the case in many in-
> stances, if only because clinical scientists often na-

ively seem to believe that the material of the trial, which is human material, is reasonably homogeneous, and that treated and untreated cases can be "matched," to use the jargon of modern clinical science. In actual fact it usually turns out to be impossible to control all the variables. (5)

And in 1964:

We are inclined to underestimate the extent of biological variation, which is such that a controlled trial is not always possible. (6)

A.B. Hill himself wrote in 1966 that the unsatisfactory outcome of many clinical trials was due to:

biological variation of the human material with which we have to deal ... Clearly our predecessors would not have got a very useful answer by applying one and the same treatment to a mixture of patients suffering from typhoid and typhus fevers before these two conditions were accurately differentiated from one another. (7)

Byron W. Brown echoed this in 1980:

statisticians know that the source of the largest uncontrolled variation in clinical experiments is not measurement variation, but the variation from patient to patient. (8)

Even such a seemingly simple trial as a comparison of mother-baby interaction immediately after birth can be plagued by the gremlins of biological variation. An analysis of sixteen reports on "early contact trials" found that the main deficiency was inadequate "definition of subjects":

For studies involving mothers' behavior toward their infants a variety of clinical (parity, neonatal birth weight, gestational age, and health status) and sociodemographic (maternal age, ethnic origin, and

31

socioeconomic status) factors could affect the outcome. (Mary Ellen Thomson, M.Sc. and M.S.Kramer, M.D., 1984)(9)

Another equally simple procedure, testing an antibiotic on infection of the incision after an abdominal operation, was found to suffer from "inadequate definition." When 45 such trials were analyzed, "six articles did not define wound infection, only twelve drew a distinction between major and minor infection, and only one, between primary and secondary infection; assessment of the extent of bacterial contamination during the operation was purely clinical in eighteen trials, microbiologic in fourteen, not mentioned in the remaining thirteen." (10)

In trials of drugs against "diseases," biological variation of the patient population and concomitant inability to "define" the subjects present even greater obstacles to a truly scientific procedure.

Although generally regarded as a problem in statistics, the current controversy about anticoagulants seems to have more basic scientific roots in the selection and classification of the patients who are the "experimental material." (R.H.Gifford, M.D, and Alvan Feinstein, M.D., 1969)(11)

Classifying patients with mental illness is still more problematic:

Research into the nature of depression and its treatment by drugs is hobbled by the fact that depressions do not constitute a single homogeneous entity. Furthermore, interpretation of reported research data in this area has been confused by a general disregard for this heterogeneity and by a lack of precision and uniformity with respect to terminology. (Charles A. Walton, Ph.D., 1968)(12)

Where diagnosis is highly subjective, and therefore imprecise, it is impossible to have homogeneous groups. Double-blind studies have been reported using anti-depressants for treating depression. The matched groups contained endogenous depressives, schizophrenics who were depressed, and neurotic depressives. When heterogeneous groups are used, the therapeutic response is so variable that the response of the treated and control groups depends too much on the random distribution of different classes of patients in them. No provision for this is made in the double-blind controlled design. (Abram Hoffer, M.D., 1967) (13)

## Sources of Heterogeneity: the Patient

Numerous possible sources of biological variation in subjects of clinical trials have been noted and discussed in the relevant literature: biographical (age, sex, race, education), historical (prior illnesses, number of pregnancies), biophysical (diet, exercise, sleep), ecological (climate, water supply, traffic pollutants, work hazards), sociopsychological (family style, relationship with doctor, desire for treatment, intelligence, persistence, religious belief), and immediate etiology of the disease (its severity, range of effects, and prior treatment). (14)

Attention should be directed, in particular, to the matter of "prior illnesses." As already noted, prior illness leaves its mark on the individual's immune system in the form of antibodies to microbial proteins associated with the earlier illness. These can and do affect all the individual's subsequent behavior and reactions. No clinical trial sample has ever been homogeneous with regard to the health histories of all its members.

An input which is difficult, if not impossible, to evaluate other than *post facto* is the varying "sensitivity" of sample members to the drug being evaluated:

In much the same way that some species of laboratory animals are superior to others for particular experiments in the laboratory, the choice of a suitable subject is often a critical matter for an investigation in man. Thus, while the best subject will tend to make the method more sensitive, unsuitable subjects may dilute the response to drugs and make the method so insensitive that it is unable to detect the particular drug action under investigation and, therefore, regardless of the activity of the drug or effectiveness of the controls, provides only a negative answer ... In studies involving subjective criteria, excessively phlegmatic subjects tend to desensitize the method by failure to react with normal sensitivity, while exceedingly neurotic and overreactive or highly suggestible patients tend to compromise the sensitivity of the method through wide swings of mood and attitude as the result both of placebo and of active medication. (Walter Modell, M.D., 1960)(15)

"Prior illness" might well be expected to affect patient sensitivity, but this also has not been systematically explored.

## Sources of Heterogeneity: the Physician

Not every physician is a good diagnostician, and their varying abilities to recognize what the patient is suffering from are a major source of sample heterogeneity. If the diagnosis is incorrect, after all, the patient may be entered in a trial for which he is quite unsuited.

Diagnostic "error" at some point shades off into legitimate and irreducible differences of medical opinion, reflecting the physician's particular area of specialization and other factors.

Hill wrote as early as 1960 that the extent of diagnostic error in the medical profession was a source of amazement to all parties. While no one was startled (he observed) when such errors were made by beginners,

it is only relatively recently that critical and courageous senior physicians and surgeons have submitted themselves to tests of their ability to agree with other equally skilled observers or with their own previous opinions, and nearly always the variability revealed has been much greater than was expected ... This variation has been found wherever it was sought. (16)

His comments have been repeated by others:

The fact that the observer's faculties and judgment enter between subject and result is obvious, but that it may substantially reduce the repeatability of the result seems to be less often appreciated. Physicians have always recognized that clinical judgments of the presence or absence, and of the severity of abnormalities, are subjective and liable to variation, at least in the hands of other members of the profession or men less qualified than themselves. The magnitude and frequency of this variability among the most skilled observers has only become apparent relatively recently as the result of investigations in many fields of medicine. In nearly every case the variation has been found to be greater than expected. (L.J.Witts, M.D., 1964) (17)

Observer bias is, of course, a well-known factor ... More subtle influences may also be at work, however. For example, a clinician's rating of one patient may depend heavily upon what other patients he has examined immediately previously; judgments have a comparative element which it is difficult to eliminate. A person who is tired may make more superficial, and hence possibly more variable, judgments than an alert fresh colleague. (F.N. Johnson, Ph.D. and S. Johnson, M.D., 1977)(18)

In 1950 six radiologists and pulmonary specialists tested their diagnostic skills on 6000 X-rays from a mass TB screening project; they differed profoundly in their interpretations, sometimes diagnosing the healthy as tuberculous and sometimes overlooking cases of pulmonary TB. In another test involving serial chest X-rays, one physician in twenty (5%)

thought the X-rays showed improvement, whereas the patient was actually deteriorating, or vice-versa. (19)

A 1964 "Bibliography on Observer Error and Variation" examined most of the studies done up until that time, including 26 studies of "clinical diagnosis," ten of "pathology and clinical chemistry," seven "anthropometric," and four "general." It covered all areas of medicine: tuberculin testing, the taking of medical histories, dental caries, X-ray interpretation, diagnosis proper (emphysema, breast cancer, blood diseases, heart diseases), biochemical analyses, autopsies, nutritional estimates, and the like. Multiple errors were found everywhere. (20)

The more ingenious and complex the diagnostic technique, the greater the probability of observer variation.

In 1967 a survey was done in Vermont of the accuracy with which six physicians could recognize throat cultures of beta-hemolytic streptococci using the standard office equipment devised for diagnosing streptococcal pharyngitis. The physicians' analyses, when compared with those of the state laboratory, were found to be wrong 33% to 75% of the time — not only failing to detect streptococci when present but mistakenly identifying negative cultures as positive. (21)

In 1979 a physician at Columbia-Presbyterian Medical Center in New York evaluated 4500 colleagues for their ability to diagnose various infectious diseases and found that half scored lower than 68%. (22)

Pathological laboratories have not done appreciably better, even though a higher standard of accuracy and uniformity might be anticipated. Often the test is not standardized, and one laboratory's definition of "normal" differs from another's. (23)

In 1956, for example, a hospital pathologist sent twenty slides of cervical biopsies, representing all stages in the development of cervical cancer, to 25 pathological laboratories for evaluation. These were not difficult or borderline slides but showed clearly the stages of development from minimal cervical atypicality to invasive cancer. Three laboratories replied that none of the slides showed cancer, one held that all thirteen showed a positive diagnosis of cancer, and the others fell in between. The author concluded that "agreement on these twenty slides is very poor" and that this sort of laboratory error may go far to explain the enormous differences in cervical cancer rates reported from different parts of the United States. (24)

The same observer variability and inaccuracy is also found in epidemiologic surveys — whether of the incidence of a disease, the birth weights of children, mortality at some given age, dietary intake, or whatever. Sound epidemiologic results are possible only if the raw data are accurate, but for decades no attention was directed to this aspect of epidemiologic investigations. In 1979 Leon Gordis for the first time called attention to the lack of control over the talents of interviewers or the quality of questionnaires, also to the absence of any effort to ensure comparability of epidemiologic data from various sources:

> No scientific discipline can be any better than its raw data ... A serious potential hazard confronting us is that, as epidemiologists, we become so enamored of increasingly sophisticated statistical techniques and data processing capabilities that we pay inadequate attention to the quality of the data obtained in our investigations — data which, in fact, become the raw material for these statistical and data-gathering methods. (25)

The impasse is due not only, or not entirely, to the differing diagnostic skills of physicians, but also to differences in clinical judgment, sometimes reflecting the differing viewpoints of the various medical specialties:

> The primary diagnosis is often quite different from the view of the internist, the surgeon, the orthopedist, or the otolaryngologist. Each selects the disease pertaining to his specialty. (E.L. DeGowin, M.D. and R.K. DeGowin, M.D., 1976) (26)

Surgeons, especially, may be prone to see a need for chirurgical intervention in almost every patient coming into their office. A notorious manifestation of this professional weakness occurred in 1935 when the American Child Health Association surveyed the tonsils of 1000 children from New York public schools. Sixty-one percent had already had their tonsils removed, and when the remaining 39% were examined by a group of physicians, just under one half were selected for tonsillectomy. The rejected children were dispatched to a different group of physicians for examination, and they again selected just under a half for tonsillectory. The procedure was repeated a third time with precisely the same outcome—about one half being selected for tonsillectory. By this time only 65 children were left in the sample:

> These subjects were not further examined because the supply of examining physicians ran out. The study showed that there was no correlation whatever between the estimate of one physician and that of another regarding the advisability of tonsillectomy. (Harry Bakwin, M.D., 1945)(27)

Even today tonsillectomy remains the third most common surgical procedure in American hospitals. The first clinical trial of its benefits was attempted in 1973 but aborted shortly thereafter when a major hospital group refused to participate. Whether or not the operation does the patient any good remains a mystery. The OTA *Background Paper* only hints delicately that tonsillectomy "is thought by many physicians to be overused." (28)

Two factors contribute to these diagnostic differences. One is the poor quality of the ordinary physician's clinical notes:

> As instruments of clinical research the routine ward notes and the machinery of hospital records are almost useless. (James Spence, M.D, 1953) (29)

> If NASA ran rockets the way most physicians run clinical records, nobody would get in those space ships. Medical knowledge is passed along like Norwegian songs in the Middle Ages, doctors singing

ballads to each other in the hospital lobby and in those show-and-tell rounds ... Doctors say, "Why do my notes have to be merged with the nurse's notes? I'm a busy man ... I don't want to know all those things." That's it, they don't want to hear about every problem of the patient. (Lawrence L. Weed, M.D., 1974) (30)

The haphazard and indisciplined collection of data resulting from the retrospective examination of case-notes seldom, if ever, produces anything of real value even though the ready availability of such case notes in general practice makes this a superficially attractive proposition. (J.E.Murphy, M.D, 1977)(31)

Poor clinical notes may reflect poor observational talent on the physician's part. In any case, the quality of the diagnosis is affected.

The second factor is the absence of applicable operational definitions which would ensure that all physicians follow the same guidelines.

Despite all the money put into academic institutions in the name of medical research, there has been very little careful categorization of patients. That information ought to have been obtained ... What I am complaining about is that there is a lack of operational definition at every level. (Alvan Feinstein, M.D., 1972)(32)

In a multi-center trial, where all physicians should adhere to the same guidelines, operational definitions would be especially important.

It is not acceptable for a clinician to assume that all, or even a substantial majority, of his colleagues adopt a common diagnostic practice: it is always mandatory for the defining criteria of the illness to be clearly, accurately, and unambiguously specified. Not only the illness, but its cure also, must be specified in this way. What one clinician may regard as a cure may either not be recognized as any cure at all by another clinician on the basis of different diagnostic criteria, or may be recorded as a partial or incomplete cure. (F.N.Johnson, Ph.D. and S. Johnson, M.D., 1977)(33)

Other sources of observer variation may contribute to the non-homogeneity of samples. For instance, instruments such as electrocardiographs from different manufacturers can yield different readings.

It may well be true that in any particular instance, the shape of an ECG as recorded is largely determined by the characteristics of the machine with which the recording was made ... The importance of the diagnostic errors that may be introduced in this manner is not always appreciated. (J.L.Meyer, M.D., 1967)(34)

The main source of error, however, is the clinical entity itself which the sample is supposed to represent. If its own contours are fuzzy, how can those of the sample be any better? Any scientific investigation must start by describing and classifying the objects or phenomena to be investigated. (35) If these phenomena are entities which have no independent existence and cannot even be described with precision, how can the clinical trial procedure possess scientific validity?

And if the sample is not "homogeneous," the results of the trial are useless, since no one knows what "disease" has actually been treated.

## Generalizability of the Sample

Not only must the patient sample be internally homogeneous, it must also accurately represent all the patients suffering from the "disease" in question. Otherwise the results obtained with the sample will not be applicable to any larger group.

This is known as "representativity" or "generalizability" of the sample.

Experiments in clinical pharmacology examine the

effect of a drug in a group of patients with a particular disease, the goal being to extend results from that sample to all patients ill with the same disease. (Theodore Greiner, M.D., 1965) (36)

Commenting on a study of epidural anesthesia vs. general anesthesia in high-risk surgical patients, Bucknam McPeek, M.D., of the Harvard Medical School, in 1987 described the factors that must be considered in determining whether or not a sample is truly representative:

Do the patients the authors describe sound like patients in our own practices? Does the general anesthesia given to the standard treatment group ... sound like the general anesthetic technique we use. Do the post-operative outcomes, the length of postoperative intubation and ventilation, and postoperative complications seem like those we observe in our own practice with high-risk surgical patients? (37)

These are the issues involved in a straightforward comparison of two types of anesthesia. When *diseases* are being compared, generalizability is even more difficult to attain.

For a patient in a clinical trial to validly "represent" the universe of patients suffering from the given "disease," he must have been selected *randomly* from that universe, meaning that every member of the universe in question had an equal chance of being included in the sample. (38) But this never occurs, and no sample is ever truly representative:

This requirement is not practical in real life, and can never be met in medical research. Since strict random procedure is impossible, errors are introduced into the study from the start, the extent of which cannot be calculated. (Theodore Greiner, M.D., 1965)(39)

The physician, after all, does not pick people at random out of a patient universe. The patients self-select themselves:

One of the most pernicious scientific delusions now prevalent in the world of medical research is the idea

41

that concepts of "random sampling" can be readily applied to clinical populations. This idea is completely vitiated by the use of patients as the "material" of clinical investigation, because a patient—unlike an agricultural field, chemical vat, or the material of any other type of experimentation — chooses the investigator, rather than vice versa ... the statistical collection of patients with that disease will be scientifically meaningless because the results cannot be extrapolated. The patients represent no one except themselves; they are a "sample" of a larger population that cannot be specified. (Alvan Feinstein, M.D., 1977) (40)

And when recruited for a trial, they are often drawn from a limited group of sources: the urban poor, prisoners, military recruits, or students — less commonly from the population at large.

The affluent classes are definitely underrepresented in clinical trials, as are those who do not know they have the condition, those whose symptoms are not very distressing, those who "do not trust doctors," and the like. The sample may be overweighted with compulsive volunteers. (41)

Children and pregnant women are usually excluded, and even women of childbearing age — and yet some conditions (rheumatoid arthritis) are disproportionately frequent among women of childbearing age.

Hospitalized patients are often tapped for entry into a clinical trial. But an element of self-selection may operate here too, as in the following example of the drug treatment of multiple sclerosis:

Before the trial all 400 patients had received the drug. Subsequently, all patients were informed that the drug's effectiveness had not been demonstrated. Some patients chose to continue taking the drug, and others did not. The patients themselves determined their therapeutic regimen, and those self-selected groups were used for the comparative study. The patients who were not receiving benefit from the drug, possibly those who were more ill, might have been more likely to stop using the drug than patients less severely disabled or in remission.

An obvious question is whether these self-selected patient groups were comparable in characteristics relevant to the progression and severity of the disease. From the information available, it was impossible to say. (William Weiss and J.M.Dambrosio, Ph.D., 1983)(42)

Hospital patients are "unrepresentative" in another sense: by definition, they have the "disease" in a more serious form, or have some concomitant "disease." This source of bias is known as "Berkson's Fallacy" in honor of Joseph Berkson, who first called attention to it in 1946. (43)

Generalizability or representativity of a sample has been described as a "complex judgmental issue which is essentially nonstatistical." It can be ensured only by employing better physicians or by radically altering the conditions of the trial. (44) Increasing the sample size or a more elaborate scheme of randomization will not help. If the method of selecting the members of the sample remains the same, the new sample is just as skewed as the old, only larger. And randomization is a technique for dividing the sample into "test" and "control" groups, not for selecting the sample in the first place.

Problems of representativity may explain why physicians complain that patients involved in clinical trials seem to differ substantially from the typical patient seen in clinical practice. (45)

A strikingly non-representative sample, one which has had a profound impact on public policy, was the one first used to measure the period of "latency" between infection with the AIDS virus and death from the pneumonia, diarrhoea, or sarcoma which are usually found in fatal cases of AIDS. The first individuals to manifest AIDS in its fatal form were a group of male homosexuals treated in a San Francisco public clinic for sexually transmitted diseases in the early 1980s. Blood samples taken from these same clients several years earlier, when they participated in a clinical trial of treatments for hepatitis, were studied for evidence of contamination with the AIDS virus. Then the average time between AIDS-virus infection and death in this group was found to be seven years. At that point American public health authorities announced that a seven-year "latency" period was applicable to the U.S. population at large, even though this sample of homosexual males had very high rates of such other venereal diseases as: syphilis, gonorrhoea, herpes, hepatitis, and others and could be expected to be far more vulnerable to the effects of HIV infection than healthier individuals. (46)

Subsequently, when the effect of AIDS virus infection in otherwise healthy persons was studied, the "latency" period was seen to be much longer than seven years. It has today been set at 14 or 15 years and promises to become even longer.

If medical authorities had been more aware of the requirement that a sample be representative, this uncertainty about the period of "latency" — which has distorted the whole public and professional discussion of AIDS — could have been avoided.

## A Therapeutic Paradox

A point not often mentioned is the paradoxical conflict between sample homogeneity and generalizabiliy. The greater the internal homogeneity of the sample, the more precisely it will distinguish treatment from no treatment, but the less representative it will be of any larger patient population. The treatment tested, therefore, will be distinguishible from the placebo but will have minimal practical application.

And, vice-versa, the less homogeneous the sample, the less capable it will be of distinguishing treatment from no treatment, but the better it will represent the real-world population of patients with the given condition. Therefore, while the benefit of any new therapy will be difficult to demonstrate, if it can be demonstrated, it will have very broad application.*

---

*A second paradox is discussed in Chapter VIII.

# IV. SAMPLE SIZE, RANDOMIZATION, STRATIFICATION

When the physician has a hypothesis to be tested and access to patients upon whom to test it, he must first decide on the size of his sample — to ensure that the outcome possesses "statistical significance."

In other words, the sample must be large enough for the conclusions to be statistically reliable. This is known as the "power" of the sample.

No general prescription for sample size exists. The rule of thumb is that it depends upon the expected magnitude of the difference in the results obtained with the new treatment as against the old, and also upon the significance level (P-value) desired. (1)

The P-value accepted in most scientific investigations is .05, meaning that the event described could occur once in twenty times purely by chance. The larger the P-value, the greater the likelihood the event could have occurred by chance. The smaller the P-value, the greater the likelihood of a causal (not a random) relationship.

Assume, for example, that an investigator has twenty patients whom he divides into two groups of ten each. Four out of ten improve in the control group, while eight out of ten improve in the test group. (2) To the outsider this treatment looks promising, but it is statistically unacceptable, since the P-value (P = .17) is larger than .05: the observed result could occur purely by chance 17 out of 100 times.

When the expected difference between the two treatments is small, larger samples are needed. When the expected difference between two treatments is large, smaller samples may be employed.

In most instances, however, the value of the "difference" (commonly represented by the Greek Δ ) is undefined. Consequently, the question of how large the sample must be cannot be answered directly. (3)

> If one realizes first of all the very crude and arbitrary nature of sample size calculations, it is clear that much ... fancy modeling and calculation may not be productive, and, in fact, may be misleading... The calculation of sample size requirements can be only a rough approximation at best. It depends on uncertain assumptions and arbitrary judgments. (Byron W. Brown, Jr., Ph.D., 1980)(4)

The classic example of a very successful trial using a very small sample was the experiment of James Lind (1716-1794) using lemons and limes to prevent scurvy. The test group consisted of two of His Majesty's seamen, while the controls were ten other seaman divided into five treatment groups. The value of the citrus fruit became evident immediately, as the ten seamen in the other groups rapidly came down with scurvy. The difference between treatment (citrus fruit) and no treatment (salt pork) was so clearcut that it became immediately evident even with tiny samples.*

By the same token, an effective treatment for cancer could be demonstrated on very small samples of terminal cases. In fact, since terminal cases always die, no control group would be needed at all.

All things being equal, the trial organizers will want to include as many patients as possible in the trial. But this conflicts with the requirement of group homogeneity. The

---

*Even so, it took the British Navy forty years to include lemons and limes in ship's stores. (T.C. Chalmers, 296).

larger the sample, the more difficult it is to ensure homogeneity. (5)

Moreover, even an apparently homogeneous sample, may contain very different individuals:

> After the population is divided into different groups, you may find that people who were old, tall, and male responded differently from those who were young, short, and female, but the distinction was being lost because everything was being lumped together. When Louis Lasagna talks about different drugs having different effects, so that one group responds, and the other does not, although both groups have the same basic disease, we are dealing with the problems that arise because any disease population contains a spectrum of different kinds of people who may respond differently. (Alvan Feinstein, M.D., 1971)(6)

Hence, the sample may have to be subdivided into homogeneous subgroups according to age, sex, race, previous illnesses, stage of disease, and the like — known as "stratification."

The sample may also be stratified in accordance with the physician's prognosis of the likely outcome for each separate patient: i.e., death or recovery, and various intermediate stages:

> In many statistically designed trials of therapy for major chronic diseases, all the patients with that disease are regularly "lumped" together for the allocation of treatment. When the results are later reported for the total group of patients, the clinician has no way of knowing whether the compared therapeutic agents had the same effects in the good prognostic risks as in the bad, or whether patients with different degrees of clinical severity responded differently. Because heterogeneous patients have been statistically managed as homogeneous, the results of an elaborate expensive trial may have little or no value for future clinical application. (Alvan Feinstein, M.D., 1977) (7)

"Randomization" of trials is seen as highly desirable. Patients are supposed to be assigned randomly to the test group or the control group, and for two reasons.

The first is to avoid biasing the outcome by, for instance, assigning patients with good prognosis to the treatment group and those with poor prognosis to the controls.

The second reason for randomization is to neutralize possible unknown contaminating variables which have not already been accounted for through stratification. (8)

The physician sometimes imagines that the mere random allocation of patients automatically ensures homogeneity of the test and control groups, in the absence of other precautionary measures. But this is to overestimate the effectiveness of the procedure. He should not assume that a group of people rounded up at the bus station can be instantly converted into suitable clinical trial material merely by allocating them randomly to the test and the control groups. Randomization is a second stage of allocation, designed to neutralize the impact of unknown variables which have not already been dealt with through stratification:

> An important part of the design is the decision about which patient characteristics that are prognostic of study outcomes should be used to define strata within which patients will be randomly assigned to treatment and which ones will be left for the act of randomization to achieve balance. (James E. Grizzle, Ph.D., 1982)(9)

Although the research community unendingly debates the relative advantages of stratification vs. randomization, and how to combine them, the ideal clinical trial would presumably involve structuring the patient population in such a way as to provide a subsample for each variable in the

---

*Some authorities, for instance, maintain that "stratified randomization" is not a true randomization technique and that, even when performed impeccably, it compromises the statistical validity of the trial outcome. (F.N.Johnson, Ph.D. and S. Johnson, M.D., 1977, 65)

disease process.* Then the members of each subsample are allocated randomly to a test group and a control group. (10) This is how the "randomized clinical trial" is presented to the American public. In fact, this ideal is seldom if ever realized.

What goes wrong?

To start with the simplest issue, randomization may be implemented more in theory than in practice. The physician may have a strong desire to incorporate a given patient in one or the other group, and when assignment is based on the flip of a coin, date of arrival, or day of the week, there are ways of ensuring that the placement is not strictly random. (11)

> The freedom of choice given to the physician in selecting patients is a source of serious error introduced by the emotional reactions of the physician. Each of us is capable of finding some way to exclude patients not likely to help in proving what we want to prove. (Theodore Greiner, M.D., 1965) (12)

> How can a physician committed to doing what he thinks is best for each patient tell a woman with breast cancer that he is choosing her treatment by something like a coin toss? How can he give up the option to make changes in treatment according to the patient's response? (Marcia Angell, M.D., 1984)(13)

> All of you are, I am sure, aware that if you favor treatment A and you have a patient with a good prognosis and the patient is going to get treatment A, and the patient doesn't want to get into the study, you are willing to sit down and spend a long time — I'm talking about your unconscious now — persuading the patient to enter the study. But if you favor treatment A and the patient looks pretty rocky, although he fulfills the written criteria of selection, and the patient says he'd rather not be in the study, you're much more easily persuaded. (Thomas C. Chalmers, M.D, 1982)(14)

Patients themselves may have a preferences for one treatment or the other and thus refuse random assignment:

> The Oxford Breast Group become involved in a study involving randomization to local excision or mastectomy initiated by the British Cancer Research Campaign and after one year found that they had entered none of the 25 eligible patients seen in that period. A review of their charts showed that most had been excluded for technical reasons ... but eight patients were ultimately asked for consent, and all eight refused. Each had strong personal preferences, three for mastectomy and five for local excision. (W.J.Mackillop,Ph.D. and Pauline Johnston,1986)(15)

Under these circumstances the scientific ideal is necessarily compromised. The results of the trial are biased.

What can be done when nonrandomized designs are considered inadequate, but randomization would be difficult because of patients' preferences for one treatment or the other? Not all problems have solutions. It simply may not be ethically possible to conduct a valid randomized clinical trial under these circumstances. (Marcia Angell, M.D., 1984)(16)

Stratification introduces a whole complex of issues. The more ramified the experiment and the larger the number of subsets, the higher the probability of diagnostic error by the admitting physician. This is particularly true of stratification according to prognosis, which is very much a matter of subjective appraisal by the physician:

> When we classify by clinic, or by sex, there is no ambiguity and little likelihood of error. However, when the criterion for classification is, say, extent of occlusion in a coronary artery as determined by angiogram, there is no absolute criterion, and there is substantial risk of error. The initial judgment, which is the basis for allocation, is made by the clinic physi-

cian, without benefit of review by higher authority. It is almost inevitable that a number of these judgments will later be found to be in error, so that low-risk patients are allocated to the high-risk stratum and vice versa. It is by no means clear, then, how the data should best be analyzed. Do we reassign those patients to the stratum specified by the review committee, or do we stay with the statistical formulation that says, "Where they were randomized is where they stay." No one has very good answers to this question, and they are mostly swept under the rug. This gap between our intention and our practice can undermine the credibility of the entire enterprise. (Paul Meier, 1981)(17)

What is definite is that, the higher the degree of stratification ("subset analysis"), the less clearcut the results of the trial, and the slighter its impact on practice. For example, clinical trials on breast cancer have:

vividly portrayed the heterogeneity of the disease and have shown that a population of such patients is composed of subgroups having different host and tumor characteristics... not all patients profit equally from the therapy. Subsets respond to a variable degree or not at all ... The dilemma is that as a result of subsetting there occurs an improvement in our comprehension of the biology of the disease, but at the same time the findings become less and less meaningful for clinical application ... Unfortunately, an inverse relationship is likely to exist between the degree of subset analysis and the clinical impact of the findings. (Bernard Fisher, M.D., 1982)(18)

This is a prime example of the malign workings of the therapeutic paradox. The more heterogeneous the sample, the harder it is to distinguish the outcome in the test group from that in the controls, and the more difficult it is to demonstrate efficacy of the new treatment. The well-conducted trial, which recognizes patient heterogeneity and accomodates it by a high degree of stratification, may yield much knowledge of the biology of the given disease but have little or no impact on practice.

But the greatest stumbling block in the path of any clinical trial, especially one demanding appreciable numbers of patients, is that the latter are always in short supply.

The more restrictive the definition of the patients to be included in the trial, the fewer the patients available. The greater the number of prognostic variables and the higher the degree of stratification, the harder it is to find patients for each subset and the larger the overall sample must be for the results obtained in each subgroup to possess statistical significance.

Some allowance must also be made for the inevitable dropping out of participants, especially during a lengthy trial. (19)

One authority has suggested that clinicians habitually overestimate the number of patients available by at least twice, and sometimes as many as ten times. (20)

The extreme difficulty of finding sufficient patients for trials has been jokingly ascribed to the workings of "Lasagna's Law" — named after its discoverer, the respected medical educator already encountered in these pages. According to this Law, "it is a worldwide experience that the supply of case material is in inverse proportion to the facilities for studying it." Or "if the supply of suitable patients available while the trial is being designed is denoted by A, then as soon as the trial is due to commence, the supply will become A/10, rising once more to A as soon as the trial ends." (21)

"Slow patient accrual" is a serious hindrance to proper conduct of the clinical trial. It has prevented some trials from being completed and has impaired the validity of others. (22) A recent survey of 39 trials found the median accrual rate to be 33 patients per year; for 24 that had reached their targeted sample size by the time of the survey, the median time required was over four years. (23) Five trials took *ten years* to reach target size. A study of cholesterol in heart disease took thirty months instead of twelve to reach the target figure;

enrolling 257 patients required screening 35,000. (24) Four large-scale American studies conducted in the past twenty years (on heart disease and hypertension) required screening almost a million contacts to locate 11,000 participants. (25)

But when a trial is extended unduly, due to inadequate patient accrual, there is a risk that the disease itself, or the patients, will have changed, so that those at the end of the trial are no longer comparable to those at the beginning:

> Every biological phenomenon is subject to minor and major cyclical changes ... to remarkable evolutionary and geophysical drifts. (Abram Hoffer, M.D., 1967)(26)

> The patient population is changing, and these changes may be quite subtle. Changes in details of treatment and changes in supportive care may also introduce subtle and unconscious biases. Diagnostic methods are changing, and we are now diagnosing diseases earlier, which makes survival look better. Survival is usually measured from the time of diagnosis. All one has to do is improve disease detection, and although nothing different has been done to affect the course of the disease, and although the patient is not living longer, it appears that there is improved survival. (Sylvan B. Green, M.D., 1982)(27)

This applies preeminently to cancer; it is being detected at an earlier stage of the disease, and the "five-year survival" rate is thus improved, even though the lives of patients have not been extended by a single day. (28) A study of colon cancer was skewed in this way by development of a diagnostic test for occult fecal blood. (29)

Curtis Meinert, of the Johns Hopkins School of Hygiene and Public Health, concluded in 1980 that "the majority of trials performed have too few patients to reach a conclusion regarding the treatments under study." (30) Marvin Zelen stated in 1982 that because sample sizes in most trials of cancer therapies were too small, i.e., possessed insufficient "power," probably only two fifths of the "positive" results reported were true positives; the remainder merely reflected the operation of chance. (31)

Lasagna's Law and its consequences can be mitigated by bringing in other hospitals and institutions — the "cooperative" or "multi-center" trial. But this leads to additional complexities of communication, timing, cost, and coordination; observer error is compounded. (32)

What is most commonly done is to alter the trial design or relax the requirements for entry into the trial, watering down the homogeneity of the sample:

> Initially the clinician will have a set of criteria which he wishes to apply when he chooses patients to include in his trial. These criteria will have been based on the theoretical requirements of the study to be undertaken and the kinds of questions being asked. Fitting criteria to patients is easy; fitting patients to criteria is quite another matter.... the design can be modified to fit the numbers available; the criteria for subject selection can be relaxed to allow the inclusion of patients previously excluded on one or more of the more stringent criteria ... All such devices have their drawbacks, of course. (F.N.Johnson, Ph.D. and S. Johnson, M.D., 1977)(33)

This necessarily means including patients who do not meet the more stringent criteria of group homogeneity. How are the late arrivals fitted in with those enrolled earlier?

> It is not satisfactory to change the trial design willy-nilly unless all the statistical implications of doing so are fully evaluated. The relaxation of selection criteria may increase the variability of therapeutic response, making statistical analysis difficult or less sensitive. (F.N.Johnson, Ph.D. and S. Johnson, M.D., 1977)(34)

These adjustments of ideal trial design to brutal realities of practice may often vitiate the results. Is the information generated truly "scientific"?

The FDA may have set itself an impossible task. "Science" is nothing if not precise. And while the design of the controlled clinical trial appears admirably precise on paper, the practice departs far from the ideal. Reproducibility is the hallmark of a truly scientific investigation, but clinical trials are often not reproducible, and not even comparable with one another.

> If the clinical analyses of one doctor and another, of one medical center and another, or of patient groups within the same medical center are to be comparable, then the populations must be identified and divided according to their pertinent clinical properties ... Without such identifications, subgroups of patients cannot validly be compared. Without the identifications, unreproducible clinical investigations are perpetuated and increased... Neither the experience of many clinicians, the reports and surveys of the medical literature, nor the data now being enthusiastically stored in computer programs have been arranged with consistent uniform classifications for differentiating precisely among clinical subgroups. Whether stored in clinician, literature, or computer, the data of one system or source often cannot be compared with those of another; physicians in one location may find they cannot rely on interpretations made elsewhere; statistical and computational analyses, therefore, yield precise but useless generalities, often inaccurate, and often valueless in application to individual patients. (Alvan Feinstein, M.D., 1976)(35)

These methodological irregularities and indeterminacies offer numerous opportunities for exercizing judgment in assembling a patient sample. Hence they may pit the physi-

---

*The vice-president of a small drug manufacturer, the Cetus Corp., told a 1989 drug-industry seminar that each year of delay in obtaining FDA approval for its new drug, *Proleukin*, added $35 million to the development cost. (Institute for Alternative Futures, December 11, 1989)

cians conducting the trial against the sponsoring manufacturer. The latter is always anxious to move forward expeditiously, even if this means cutting methodologic corners.* Since it is probably footing the bill, its preferences carry weight.

Clinical trials are extremely expensive, accounting for one quarter of a new drug's $150-$200 million development costs, and the greater the number of participants, the greater the expense. This is always in the mind of the sponsor and leads to a strong preference for smaller samples. (36)

The risk that the sample may be too small, and thus lose its representativity, may be the least of the sponsor's concerns.

One drug-company representative gave the following advice to a gathering of physicians, showing how samples are often assembled in practice:

> The most essential qualification of an investigator is that he should have, or have access to, an appropriate number of suitable patients ... The supply of patients is a totally different matter. It is governed by Lasagna's Law ... What causes the curious disappearance of suitable patients as soon as we initiate a clinical trial? Usually we do. By "we" I mean medical advisors in the industry, or anyone else who undertakes the detailed planning of a trial. In the interests of safety, ethical considerations, and accepted standards of design, we stipulate patient selection criteria that exclude a high proportion of the available population ... Everyone who writes about the design of clinical trials contributes to the operation of Lasagna's Law by insisting upon certain design criteria such as precision of diagnosis, homogeneity of groups, comparability of groups, and occasionally even matched pairs of patients. Good statistics cannot validate a poorly designed test, but neither can elaborate statistics compensate for inadequate amounts of patients, however well-designed or well-executed the trial may be. I do not dispute the desirability of Professor Wilson's

design requirements, and, when we are dealing with a very common disease entity, they may be met in full. When dealing with uncommon conditions, some compromises must be accepted. It is no use writing a perfect protocol for a trial that cannot be carried out. Comparability of groups is by far the most important factor in determining the validity of a clinical trial, and the easy way to achieve comparability is to use a lot of patients. That is why Lasagna's Law is such a serious bugbear...

If you have to choose between homogeneity and [representativity], don't compromise with [representativity]. Relax your acceptance criteria, and resort to stratified randomization. You may, for example, accept out-patients as well as in-patients provided that you allocate the same number of each to each group. In the same way, if specifying "classical rheumatoid arthritis" according to ARA criteria provides too few patients, you may have to include the "definite" and even the "probable" categories as well. This type of compromise contains a hidden bonus: the less diagnostically definite cases of disease usually include those of recent onset who may be more responsive to treatment. This improves the sensitivity of the experiment.

Third, don't divide your patients into more groups than is absolutely necessary.

Fourth, if formal patient consent is to be sought, don't make it harder than necessary for the investigator to get it.

Fifthly, don't insist upon the exclusion of certain categories of patients unless it is really essential. If a drug causes damage to the gastrointestinal mucosa of experimental animals, it would seem at first sight mandatory to exclude patients with a history of peptic ulceration, but the argument loses much of its validity if the alternative treatments for the patient's condition are aspirin, phenylbutazone, indomethacin, and corticosteroids. Even when animal studies suggest possible teratogenicity, it may still be quite proper to include married women of childbearing age provided they are taking oral contraceptives. One of our investigators used to send young women whom he wished to include in a clinical trial to see his wife who ran the family planning clinic.

Much could be said about investigators and patients, but I will conclude by reemphasizing that they are the essential components of clinical investigation. There are rarely enough of either, but the investigator usually brings his patients with him. So when you have selected your investigator, do try not to exclude nine-tenths of his patients by prohibitively strict selection criteria ... (J.A.L.Gorringe, M.D., 1970)(37)

This is the voice of reality! In the contest between economic and scientific stringencies, the economic one will generally win. The quick and dirty sample is put together, and the trial proceeds.

# V.  MEASURING THE VARIABLES. DEFINING CURE

The clinical trial process necessitates comparisons between the patient's initial and final states as well as between the test group and the control group. And comparisons demand measurement.

But measuring the patient's initial state of health, his final state, and the changes that occur during sickness and cure is not a self-evident procedure.

## What Is To Be Measured And How?

In the ordinary practice of medicine the physician decides whether or not the patient is cured merely by observing and asking questions. At some point they both agree that the patient "feels better" or "feels well," and that is the end of it. This method of judging, however, is not widely employed in clinical trials. It is thought to be excessively subjective, with a wide margin of error due to the varying observational talents of physicians and their differing understanding of "feeling better" or "feeling well."

Instead, the physician seeks characteristics of the disease process which truly and uniquely define it and which yield an objective evaluation of the patient's clinical state. These may be symptoms, biochemical changes, or pathological alterations.

Until the late nineteenth century the physician's knowledge was mostly symptomatic. He relied for diagnosis on what he could observe with his own senses and what he could

59

elicit from the patient by questioning. Today, with so many biochemical, radiographic, and pathological techniques available, preference is given to these alternative sources of clinical knowledge, while the patient's often ambiguous symptoms have fallen somewhat into disfavor.

But the physician's traditional skill at observing symptoms still has a role to play, in both physical and mental disease. Indeed, the latter can rarely be defined other than symptomatically.

> It is not, for example, easy to distinguish depression from anxiety, and the use of a diagnostic category called "anxiety-depression" does little to solve the problem. In such cases it is essential that the clinician undertaking a trial not simply ignore the matter, leaving the question of the accurate diagnosis of the illness to the caprice of his various colleagues who are involved in the trial. (F.N.Johnson, Ph.D. and S. Johnson, M.D., 1977)(1)

> When I sat in on one of the committees involved in drawing up the clinical research guidelines for the FDA, some of these issues were glossed over, particularly the problem of diagnosis in psychiatric disorders. This would include such questions as the following: How much anxiety is necessary? What criteria should be used to include a patient in a trial? ... much concern was expressed about freezing this set of guidelines. (Gerald L. Klerman, M.D., 1971)(2)

He always hopes that one or several specific symptoms will be clearly linked to the disease in question, with changes in these symptoms revealing changes in the disease:

> The symptoms of the illness must be carefully and objectively specified and classified. It is only rarely that an illness can be defined in terms of a single symptom: it is more often the case that several symptoms are definitive of the condition. These must be listed and ranked in order of importance so that a decision may be made as to which, if any, are to be

disregarded in assessing treatment outcome. (F.N.Johnson, Ph.D. and S. Johnson, M.D., 1977)(3)

Thus anorexia, jaundice, and a tender liver often indicate infectious hepatitis; wheezing and coughing up of blood often point to lung cancer; skin lesions, arthritis, and nephritis may indicate the autoimmune disease, lupus erythematosus, etc., and as these alter, so does the "underlying disease" in question. (4)

The patient's "overall index of well-being" is sometimes part of the anamnesis:

Such global ratings necessarily embody a large subjective component and will therefore be likely to vary from clinician to clinician. Given, however, that they are clinically relevant measures (whether or not they should be is, of course, another question), it is reasonable that they should be included in the symptom checklist. (F.N.Johnson, Ph.D. and S. Johnson, M.D., 1977)(5)

But how is subjectivity avoided? How, for instance, does the physician measure pain?

A clinician could measure height, blood pressure, urinary volume, and cardiac output, but how could he measure headache, angina pectoris, dysuria, or anxiety? What could a clinician possibly do to measure all of the subjective sensations, qualitative signs, and personal reactions that were inevitable parts of the data noted in clinical observation? (Alvan Feinstein, M.D., 1976)(6)

As I remember the Eastern Solid Tumor Chemotherapy Group meeting, preparing the check sheets on which the clinical data were to be recorded was especially trying because defining the entries was so difficult. It was much easier to define the white counts. Much more time was spent in group discussions of how to record clinical data. (Thomas C. Chalmers, M.D., 1971)(7)

One solution is to objectify the symptoms, but this is more difficult than might at first appear.

The Karnofsky Scale, for instance, is widely employed to assess the functional state of persons with cancer, its three main categories being: (1) ability to work, (2) ability to carry on normal activities, and (3) ability to care for oneself. One would expect the grading of this test to be virtually automatic, but when two pairs of physicians were asked to evaluate 60 patients according to the Karnofsky Scale, agreement between them was only 34% for one pair and 29% for the other. (8)

> One way in which the problem of interobserver variability may be overcome is by arranging for all recordings to be done by instruments which print out the appropriate measurement in clear and unequivocal numerical terms. This is not, however, possible for many clinically important symptoms, and so the issue of measurement reliability cannot be avoided. (F.N.Johnson, Ph.D. and S. Johnson, M.D., 1977)(9)

When patients are offered a three- or four-point scale ("none," "slight," "definite," "unbearable," etc.), they will usually pick the middle term. If additional categories are added, the patient simply becomes confused. (10) An attempt to evaluate the pain of an arthritic joint by subjecting it to "firm pressure" and recording the response, was not reproducible by different observers. (11)

For all these reasons the relatively "soft" symptoms recede into the background as sources of important clinical information, in favor of the more readily quantifiable results of laboratory tests. This reflects Kelvin's dictum: "When you cannot express it in numbers, your knowledge is of a meager and unsatisfactory kind."

Today the major scientific variables used in clinical strategy often come from patients only indirectly; patients provide the substances that yield the data discerned from examinations in the laboratory. The scientific aspects of modern medical care are therefore often focused more on the patient's laboratory identification as a diseased organism than on his bedside identity as a sick person. (Alvan Feinstein, M.D., 1976)(12)

The physician would like to have one or two readily quantifiable data, known as "endpoints" or "variates" — survival time, white blood count, a surgical complication, a fatal surgical complication, and the like — which yield a reliable indication of the patient's status. (13)

Over the years committees have developed clinical indexes and criteria of endpoints for the therapy of asthma, cerebrovascular accidents, congestive heart failure, coronary artery disease, hay fever, leukemia, lung disease, multiple myeloma, rheumatic fever, rheumatoid arthritis, thyrotoxicosis, and others. These, however, have not been systematically tested in practice,

And, for ... many other major diseases, there still remains the problem that appropriate therapeutic indexes and criteria, if existing, are not used, and if absent, are not contemplated and developed. (Alvan Feinstein, M.D., 1976)(14)

The preference for "objective" parameters of sickness and health is strengthened by the availability of instruments capable of performing physiological measurements accurately and instantaneously on large numbers of people. A value which can be readily measured will be favored by the organizers of clinical trials. But this involves the danger that a parameter only marginally relevant to the disease process will be selected merely because it is readily accessible.

A drop in the erythrocyte sedimentation rate, for example, which is easy to measure, usually signifies clinical improvement in rheumatoid arthritis, but some patients improve even when the reading remains elevated. (15) How, then, is clinical improvement in rheumatoid arthritis to be determined?

The identification of blood cholesterol levels with coronary artery disease was reinforced by the availability of a simple technique for measuring cholesterol. Formerly the ratio of the various fatty acids in a blood sample — some "saturated" and some "unsaturated" — had to be calculated by the "million monkey method," measuring peaks on a gas-liquid chromatograph by hand. In the late 1960s, however, this process was automated, and the medical students who had earned spending money tracing these peaks had to seek other sources of income. (16)

Administration of a chemical drug to lower the cholesterol, and thus prevent coronary artery disease, was the next logical step, and the "antihyperlipidemic" medicines were developed for this purpose.

However rational this approach may have seemed, the results were disappointing. There turned out to be a divergence between the "chemical efficacy" of this treatment and its "therapeutic efficacy." Even when the selected parameter (fatty acids in the blood) registered improvement, the patient's status remained unchanged or even deteriorated. The physician is so advised by the "package insert":

It must be understood that there is no evidence that use of any lipid-altering agent will be beneficial in preventing death from coronary artery disease. (17)

Antihyperlipidemic agents are still used to treat and prevent coronary artery disease, and have been licensed by the FDA for this purpose, but they confer no benefit.

Patients with myocardial infarction are sometimes given anti-arrhythmic agents to stabilize and regularize the heartbeat; but even when the heartbeat is stabilized, mortality is identical to what it would have been in the absence of medication. (18)

Long-acting nitrites are prescribed for angina pectoris, and have been so prescribed for more than a century. But the ability of these drugs to change the ECG, dilate the coronary arteries, or increase coronary blood flow does not make them effective in treating angina pectoris. Dilatation of the normal artery, for example, does not mean that more blood is also flowing through the calcified artery, and could mean that less blood is flowing through the calcified artery. Furthermore, there is little correlation between changes in the cardiogram and the occurrence of angina pectoris. (19) Five to ten percent of angina pectoris cases have anatomically normal coronary arteries (known as "atypical angina").(20)

The same comment can be made about the use of oral hypoglycemic medicines in diabetes. The disease is marked by an elevated blood-sugar level — again a factor which can readily be measured, and its reduction was thought to be tantamount to cure.

Tolbutamide (*Orinase*) and chlorpropamide (*Diabinase*) were developed for this purpose. But the outcome did not justify the initial assumption. Here, too, the drug's chemical efficacy differed from its therapeutic efficacy. Blood sugar levels declined, but the patients still died. The physician is advised by the package insert:

> it should be recognized that controlling the blood glucose in noninsulin-dependent diabetes has not been definitely established to be effective in preventing the long-term cardiovascular or neural complications of diabetes. (21)

These all illustrate one more paradox of the clinical trial procedure. The value which can be measured may not be relevant, while the value which is relevant may not be "objectively" measurable.

What medicine needs, in Feinstein's view, is to endow the observation of symptomatic phenomena with the rigor of "objective" instrumental measurements by developing and applying "operational definitions." This would yield a "clinical nosology" representing the consensus of physicians on the definition of the signs and symptoms specific to each disease. (22)

> The methods of an experiment must be adapted to the material. The methods of laboratory research provide neither the technology nor the judgment for the *clinical*

study of people ...Clinicians use excellent techniques for observing and studying animals, or the parts of a person as the entities of the laboratory, but inadequate techniques for studying a whole person as the human entity at the bedside. (Alvan Feinstein, M.D., 1976)(23)

Instead of zealously seeking dimensional measurement for symptoms, signs, and other human properties that cannot be dimensionally measured with precision or convenience, clinicians must seek ways of improving the value of their own clinical descriptions of these entities. (Alvan Feinstein, M.D, 1976)(24)

But this would require the physician to become a good observer — a talent which is often lacking in today's medical profession:

The clinical examination of patients is frequently dismissed as unreliable because the data are not always reproducible. Yet the unreliability is often attributable to the examiner, not the patient. (Alvan Feinstein, M.D, 1976)(25)

## "Baseline" Values

Once the parameter has been selected, the physician needs what is called a "baseline" value against which to measure deviations. What is the value of this parameter in health, and how does it vary during disease?

Without this knowledge the physician cannot determine if the medication has made any difference.

The baseline value means the "normal" value, and defining "normality" is always a puzzle.

In the past, baseline values were obtained by observing what happened in untreated cases or by analyzing the historical record. But information on the "natural history" of diseases is not readily available today when few patients are willing to forego treatment merely to add to society's store of medical knowledge. Furthermore, many diseases (syphilis, tuberculosis, and scarlet fever come to mind) have under-gone modification due to acquisition of herd immunity by the subject populations. Baseline values cannot be taken from the historical record but must be updated. (26)

And how are baseline parameters determined in the case of a "new" disease? Norbert Wiener once pointed out that any new disease comes to the profession's attention because of a series of fatalities. Diagnostic techniques are then devised which enable the physician to identify the condition at an earlier stage when, in many cases, it is mild and self-limiting.

For these reasons, baseline values are not simply there, ready-made for the physician's taking. They must be *established*, and this is the object of the most intense negotiation between the drug manufacturer (desiring a baseline which will show his new drug to the greatest advantage) and the FDA. One officer of that agency reported:

> Requirements for representative baseline values prior to drug administration frequently provoke a battle that involves the most pontifical of moral rhetoric. (J. Marian Bryant, M.D., 1972)(27)

## The Definition of Cure

The physician cannot merely ask the patient if he or she feels better, but must seek an "objective" criterion of cure. This, however, is unexpectedly complicated. Even the most apparently straightforward clinical trial, say, a study of a new antibiotic in pneumonia, may be excessively difficult to evaluate:

> You are treating two patients with bacteriologically proven pneumococcal lobar pneumonia. Both patient X and patient Y are men, of the same age, and without such complications as diabetes or kidney or heart disease. X is given the latest wonder drug, Miracle-cillin, and Y receives penicillin.

The white blood count of X is 12,000 per cubic mm.; for Y 16,000. Is one sicker than the other? Can you quantitate the pulmonic involvement on X ray? Patient X has had symptoms for two days. Patient Y for three. Are they truly comparable cases? It would be as rare as finding matching fingerprints to find two patients with absolutely identical clinical signs, symptoms, and laboratory data. We have no way of measuring "resistance." We cannot even measure the nutritional state accurately. At any rate, we treat X and Y. Three days later X's chest is unclear, but the white cell count is still elevated; Y's X-ray still shows fuzzy shadows, but his laboratory tests have become normal. How would you judge — computer notwithstanding — whether his response is good, fair, or poor? Were the cases comparable to begin with? Let us not forget that there is always a strong subjective element in research.

I think you can see that even in a field as relatively objective as antibiotic therapy there are problems of clinical evalation. Think how much more complex the situation is for analgesics or tranquilizers, for example. It is hard enough for the clinician at the bedside to make a judgment; it is harder still for the reader to make a judgment of the literature.

I have no easy solution to the problem except to plead for understanding. (S.O.Waife, M.D., 1968)(28)

In one antibiotic trial patients were reported "cured" even though they had swollen glands persisting for weeks. What if another medicine had cured them without the legacy of swollen glands? (29)

Mental illnesses present their usual intractable dilemmas:

We really cannot define what we mean by efficacy in regard to the psychotropic drugs. (Elmer Gardner, M.D., 1971) (30)

Even though the FDA's task is to evaluate drug "efficacy," no definition of "efficacy" exists. (31)

One little-discussed possibility is that the existing treatment may be positively harmful — so that its mere cessation would bring benefit:

> it is important that the *standard treatments themselves* should be shown to be better than placebo and safe when compared with complications resulting from the disease itself [stress added]. (Michael B. Bracken, M.D, 1987)(32)

That a standard treatment might be more harmful than doing nothing at all is not a purely hypothetical possibility. A 1956 study of surgery and radiation therapy in cancer concluded that:

> untreated cases are perhaps longer-lived than the treated cases ... for not only is there complete uncertainty of the efficacy of cancer treatment today, but there is also the possibility that survival tendency is less with treatment. It is most likely that, in terms of life expectancy, the chance of survival is no better with than without treatment, and there is the possibility that treatment may make the survival time of cancer cases less. (Hardin B. Jones, Ph.D., 1956)(33)

In 1990 a German biostatistiacian who had worked for a decade as a favored associate on cancer chemotherapy projects published a devastating critique of this mode of treatment, claiming that chemotherapy does not extend life to any appreciable extent and expressing doubt that it even improves the patient's quality of life. The whole purpose of chemotherapy — to shrink the tumor — is misguided according to Ulrich Abel, since shrunken tumors nearly inevitable rebound and become more deadly. In fact, patients in whom chemotherapy does not affect tumor size tend to live longer. (34)

The above strictures against the surgical, radiation, and chemotherapeutic treatment of cancer are doubtless true, in view of the steady rise in cancer incidence and mortality in

Western societies. And yet new cancer treatments are often measured against existing ones.

These are all problems of clinical judgment and should be dealt with in that context. But the physician's (subjective!) judgment is not trusted, and the clinical trial aims to minimize its scope. Investigators continue their relentless search for the objective parameter which yields the truth about the patient's changed condition:

> To avoid this type of messy imprecision, the statistician opts for the neatness of analyzing a single univariate response; the investigator agrees; and another clinical trial produces simplistic results that have little pertinence to the complex world of reality. (Alvan Feinstein, M.D., 1977)(35)

# VI.  THE DOUBLE-BLIND PROCEDURE. CONDUCT OF THE CLINICAL TRIAL

In contrast to earlier medical history, when the physician was valued for his ability to observe, the twentieth century asserts that truth is attained by depriving the doctor of vision. The so-called "double-blind" trial, where neither doctor nor patient know what the latter is receiving, has been devised as a technique which supposedly allows truth to shine forth by removing the shackles of prejudice and preconception.

Two objections may be made to the concept of "blinding."

First, it is a theoretical construction which has never been calibrated or subjected to experimental verification. (1) It is assumed to compensate for bias in the observer and faith in the patient, but its efficacy for these purposes has never been demonstrated by an empirical test. *Quis custodiet ipsos custodes?*\*

Second, as so often occurs in clinical trials, the practice departs from the theory. Physicians and patients become "unblinded" rather often — far more so than anyone cares to admit:

It is easy enough to include in the clinical trial protocol the requirement that neither the patient nor the person responsible for assessing clinical response (doctor, nurse, or other personnel) should, either before or

---

\*"Who shall guard the guards themselves?"

during the trial, be aware of which medication is being prescribed at any given time to an identified patient. It is less easy to ensure that this requirement is met and maintained. Many reports have appeared outlining the ways in which blindness is broken... this ideal is difficult to establish and maintain. (F.N.Johnson, Ph.D. and S. Johnson, M.D., 1977)(2)

Patients, after all, want to know what is happening to them, and so do their physicians, nurses, and family members. Those concerned make every conceivable effort to distinguish medicine from placebo:

It is doubtful if more than a small proportion of these experiments are really blind. Hardly ever does the design of the study ensure that at no time will the code be broken by doctor or nurse observers. In many psychiatric wards there is a tradition among nurses which ensures that every attempt will be made to break the code. Nurses are no worse than doctors and, like doctors, they also have ethical problems about giving their patients a placebo. They will chew, taste, swallow the tablets, suspend them in water, pound them with a hammer, throw them against the wall, and stamp on them. They will study the fluid characteristics of the coded liquid in syringes and see how it mixes with blood which may flow back into the barrel. It seems the double-blind not only reduces faith to an undesirably low level, but brings out petty larceny in all of us. (Abram Hoffer, M.D., 1967)(3)

The code may be broken by the pharmacist. Since Medicare, Medicaid, and insurance programs usually refuse to underwrite prescriptions of inert substances, the patient may learn he is in the control group when the pharmacist asks him to pay for his "medication." (4)

Sometimes the difference in outcome is too revealing. In a study of phenylpropanolamine vs. placebo to control mild obesity, 74% of placebo participants and 43% of those on the active medication guessed their treatment correctly. The appetite control for which the phenylpropanolamine was administered in the first place gave it away. (5)

A trial of lithium carbonate to prevent or control mood swings was deciphered by both nurses and the patients' relatives:

> Nurses proved able to detect patients on active medication, though this ability varied in degree from nurse to nurse and the guesses were, in general, more accurate if the patient had been in the trial for fifteen months or more, rather than for shorter periods. The patients' relatives were extraordinarily perceptive and readily detected the use of active medication ... (F.N.Johnson, Ph.D. and S. Johnson, M.D., 1977)(6)

If the two treatments differ in their appearance or mode of administration, blindness is impossible to maintain. In one large study of heart disease (the Multiple Risk Factor Intervention Trial) the experimental group received intensive counseling while the control group received none, making it quite clear who was in which group. (7)

In a drug trial the two pills may taste different: "although the capsules were indeed identical, the difference in the contents was childishly obvious." (8) The suggestion has even been made that, before characterizing a drug trial as "double-blind," authors supply evidence that a "taste committee" has certified the contents of the different capsules to be indistinguishible. (9)

Sometimes the medication is betrayed by side-effects or toxicities. (10) Or the absence of adverse reactions reveals the placebo. (11) The requirement that patients give "informed consent" to inclusion in therapeutic trials, involving an enumeration of possible side effects, enables them to recognize reactions when they occur; they may then withdraw from the trial and are, in any case, no longer blinded. (12)

Thus, an undetermined proportion of supposedly "blind" trials are not really "blind" at all. To ascertain the precise extent of this undetermined proportion would be impossible, however, since the fact is not likely to be publicized.

One wag has urged that the defects of the double-blind procedure be remedied by more of the same: physician and patient should not know who receives the drug and who the placebo, the druggist should not know what medicine he is prescribing, and the statistician should not know which set of figures applies to which group of patients. This would be called the "quadruple blind" experiment! (13)

A better solution would simply be to recognize that blindness, like other aspects of the controlled clinical trial, is to a large degree mythical — a utopian ideal which is unrealizable in practice. The method could then be reconstructed to allow the physician once again to develop and apply his powers of observation.

In any case, not all trials are blinded. For example, of 755 funded by the National Institutes of Health in 1975, only 114 were double-blind in design. (14)

A major obstacle to success in the controlled clinical trial is its administrative complexity:

> It is probably not an exaggeration to say that a trial is one-tenth medicine and nine-tenths bureaucracy... It takes time to make recordings of clinical response and the total time commitment is a direct function of the number of measures included in the study, the recording time for each, and the frequency with which such measures are obtained throughout the trial period. Total time may be reduced by a decrease in any or all of these, the precise balance depending both upon the kind of information required from the trial and the available resources of the trial team. It is all too easy to overestimate the amount of time which people are prepared to spend in repetitive activities over an extended period, and the wise trial designer will not only make moderate demands in this direction, but will also take special note of the problems involved in obtaining measurements at weekends, public holidays, staff holiday periods, at night, at mealtimes, and so on. (F.N.Johnson, Ph.D. and S. Johnson, M.D., 1977)(15)

The administrative burden grows heavier as the trial design becomes more complex, as more centers participate, as the number of patients grows larger, and as trial groups become more stratified. (16) The longer the trial, the more its outcome depends upon retaining staff familiar with the project history, and the greater the likelihood that the data and the records will become confused. (17) There is real danger that the purpose of the trial will be undermined and the data vitiated.

Finally, the value of the clinical trial may be undermined by slipshod or dishonest execution. Defects of implementation — ranging from lack of attention to trial protocols and inadequate record-keeping to the wholesale fabrication of data — are discovered whenever a search for them is made.

Some highlights from FDA history since adoption of the Kefauver-Harris Amendments will be instructive.

In 1967 FDA Commissioner James Goddard established a six-person Scientific Investigation Group headed by Frances O. Kelsey, M.D. (the medical officer who prevented thalidomide from being marketed in the United States) to check New Drug Applications for completeness and accuracy.*The group found that five of the first 25 applications investigated contained enough defects to warrant issuing a reprimand or barring the physicians from further investigations. Most cases involved failure to keep or provide adequate records. The group also investigated fifty physicians engaged in clinical trials and found that sixteen had supplied false data on drugs to the sponsoring companies and to the government. (18)

One of them, an associate professor of medicine at Tulane, was later indicted by a Louisiana grand jury for submitting two reports, to two companies, on the same trial.

---

*"New Drug Application" (NDA) is the official name for the drug company's request to market a new pharmacological entity.

The Kinslow Commission, also appointed by Goddard, issued a report at this time assailing the drug industry for the poor quality of its clinical research and failure to observe the requirements of the controlled trial. (19)

In 1969 R.H.Gifford, M.D. and Alvan Feinstein, M.D. studied 32 trials of anticoagulent drugs in acute myocardial infarction. Only one fourth provided precise diagnostic criteria of the condition studied; only three fourths employed a control group; in only four trials were patients allocated randomly to treatment and control groups, and only one of the studies was double-blind. (20)

In 1969 Dale Console, M.D., testified before a committee of Congress about his almost seven years as associate medical director and medical director of E.R.Squibb & Sons:

These are some of the things [the medical director] must learn to rationalize.

He must learn the many ways to deceive the FDA and, failing in this, how to seduce, manipulate, or threaten the physician assigned to the New Drug Application into approving it even if it is incomplete.

He must learn that anything that helps to sell a drug is valid, even if it is supported by the crudest testimonials, while anything that decreases sales must be suppressed, distorted, and rejected because it is not absolutely conclusive proof.

He must learn to word a warning statement so it will appear to be an inducement to use the drug rather than a warning of the dangers inherent in its use ...

He will find himself squeezed between businessmen who will sell anything and justify it on the basis that doctors ask for it, and doctors who demand products they have been taught to want through advertising and promotion schemes contrived by businessmen. If he can absorb all this and more, and still maintain any sensibilities, he will learn the true meaning of loneliness and alienation. (21)

Herbert Ley, M.D., former FDA Commissioner, stated in 1970: "Between 1963 and the period from '66 to '70, both the FDA and industry were learning to live with the requirements of the new law. It is hard for an outsider to realize the quality deficiencies in some applications from firms that have been processed over this seven-year period." (22)

J. Marion Bryant, M.D., an FDA officer during the period in question, gave a front-line description of his own interaction with drug-company employees:

> Work with NDA material makes statistics appear in another guise: that of one of the more creative of the arts, with the computer as its scapegoat. Validity of input data seems to be regarded as not necessarily essential. In the presence or absence of complete data, the statistical description sometimes misrepresented as proof is assisted by a sophisticated type of clairvoyance technically known as "plugging." ... Gross deficiencies are almost uniformly encountered in submitted material ..."raw data" are either unavailable or appallingly deficient. In addition, interpretations by investigators and sponsors alike, at times, appear distinctly at odds with the data — so much so as to suggest the practice of magic rather than that of science.... Assertions of that sort often utilize such fallacies of rhetoric, in support of nonexistent or inadequate data, as might cause Socrates to weep. Expositions of pharmacologic mechanism are replete with speculative rationalizations stated as conclusions but unsupported by necessary proof. The distinction between theory and fact is sometimes more obscured than a view of Staten Island from the Battery by Manhattan smog. (23)

In 1972 the FDA conducted a survey of 155 clinical investigations: 74% failed to comply with one or more provisions of the law and the regulations, 50% failed to keep accurate records of the amount of drugs received from the sponsor and distributed to test subjects, 28% failed to adhere to the study protocol (which should have, but did not, invalidate the whole trial), 23% failed to maintain records which accurately reflected the condition of the patient before, during, and after the study, 22% did not retain case records as required, and 12% failed to supervise the study properly. (24)

Then, at the request of the General Accounting Office, the FDA inspected a sample of 35 sponsor/investigators from the list of 1973 New Drug Applications; all 35 had failed to comply with one or more of the FDA's regulations. In July, 1976, the General Accounting Office stated, in a detailed report on the FDA:

> The Food and Drug Administration has neither adequately monitored new drug tests nor adequately enforced compliance with testing requirements. Consequently, it lacks assurance (1) that the thousands of human subjects used in such tests annually are protected from unnecessary hazards of new drugs or (2) that the test data used in deciding whether to approve new drugs for marketing are accurate and reliable. (25)

FDA Commissioner Alexander Schmidt admitted at the time: "What's been most disturbing is the frank falsification of data. We have found that too often." (26)

The Special Committee on Internal Pollution — an ad hoc group with distinguished membership appointed in the United Kingdom — reported in 1975:

> Clinical trials of new compounds conducted by doctors are a shambles. Twenty percent of doctors doing such trials in the United States in 1973 whose work was spot-checked by the Food and Drug Administration were found guilty of a range of unethical practices, including wrong doses and falsifying records. Indeed, of all the reports submitted, the trial had not been carried out at all in about one third of them, in a third the established protocol had not been followed, and in only a third were the results of any scientific value. (27)

In 1989, Martin F. Shapiro, M.D. and Robert P. Charrow, J.D. reported on 1955 FDA audits of trials between 1977 and 1988 and found "serious deficiencies" in 11%. Four types of misconduct were noted:

> (1) Deliberate "fudging" or "drylabbing" of data, apparently for purposes of academic advancement; (2) deliberate deceit, apparently for economic gain (fraud); (3) arrogant disregard of protocols; and (4) unintentional errors due to an investigator's lack of experience or competence. (28)

*One quarter* of the trials failed to adhere to the protocol, and *one quarter* kept inaccurate records or refused to make records available (the two categories often overlapped). There was no decline in the incidence of these types of misconduct during the period under study.

A subcategory of inadequate record-keeping is the non-reporting of concomitant therapy which might interfere with evaluation of the drug being tested. Alan B. Lisook, M.D., Chief of the FDA Clinical Investigations Branch, told a 1989 European Symposium on Good Clinical Practice:

> We have found patients being studied for relief of arthritis pain by non-steroidal anti-inflammatory drugs to have been taking glucocorticoids, and those on a study of antidepressants to be taking anxiolytics, etc. We are not too concerned if these confounding drugs are reported, but often they are not. (29)

Thus, in more than one case out of four the data submitted to the FDA had little or no relationship to the actual clinical findings, i.e., were essentially invented out of whole cloth (known to the FDA as "graphite data"). (30) States Alan Lisook:

> I consider the audit of data, i.e., the comparison of documents submitted to FDA with data on site which might support the veracity of those documents, to be of paramount importance. (31)

But it may sometimes be difficult to locate these "data on site." Alan Lisook described the FDA's problems in this respect:

> It is amazing how many times what we refer to as the *Andrea Doria* phenomenon occurs. Here are some of the reasons why records were not available:
>
> "They were destroyed in a fire."
> "They were destroyed in a flood."
> "They were destroyed in a hurricane."
> "They were destroyed in an earthquake."
> "They were dropped in a sewer and had to be destroyed because of the stench."
> "They were lost in a boating accident."
> "My office was burglarized (and/or vandalized)."
> "The hospital closed, and the records were lost."
> "They were lost in the mail."
> "The mover threw them out."
> "My father-in-law threw them out."
>
> Under the same *Andrea Doria* phenomenon are horrible things which happen to investigators which cause unreliable data to be submitted:
>
> Co-Investigators dead or missing
> Clinical Lab Technician dead or missing.
> Office Nurse dead or missing.
> The Nurse or Resident did it, and I didn't know (subgroup: "They were out to get me").

Frightful examples of dishonesty, fraud, negligence, and other kinds of wrongdoing in clinical trials have been staple fare for readers of the daily press since the 1970s, when Congressional committees and subcommittees renewed their interest in this topic.

A few typical examples may be cited.

In 1976 the General Accounting Office found that trials of a drug designed to prevent rejection of kidney transplants led to 85 deaths in the 650 patients participating; none of these deaths were reported to the FDA. (32)

In 1978 FDA Commissioner Donald Kennedy testified at a Hearing of the Senate Health Subcommittee about audits of thirteen physicians who were doing drug trials for 48 major manufacturers, including Roche Laboratories, Bristol-Myers, McNeil Laboratories, and Endo Laboratories. Describing the findings as "horrible" and "inconceivable," Kennedy told of reports on patients who did not exist, never got the drug, never gave informed consent to being tested, did not have the disease which the drug was supposed to treat, or were administered dangerously high doses. One M.D. investigator told the FDA that a friend was conducting his trial on a muscle relaxant; halfway through the trial the FDA contact read in the daily press that the friend had died, but the doctor continued to report his friend's results. Another doctor was supposedly testing a Roche Laboratories sedative on eleven patients in a VA Hospital; charts showed that only one actually got the drug; halfway through the test two patients died; none of this information was told to the FDA, as Roche officials "reinterpreted and changed the data" (according to the FDA). (33)

The physicians were being paid handsomely for their work — between $24,000 and $106,000 for a trial lasting up to one year. "Their reports invariably were optimistic," stated Commissioner Kennedy, "sometimes to the point of inciting suspicion within the sponsoring firm."

Senator Edward Kennedy, conducting this hearing, noted that if only 10% of the data from ongoing clinical trials is defective, the problem is enormous. "When you consider the potential cumulative effect of faulty animal data coupled with faulty human data, you have the elements of a regulatory nightmare." (34)

But as we have already seen, the figure is not 10% but perhaps 25%. We are undoubtedly in the midst of a "regulatory nightmare," although no one has called attention to it.

In 1979 the Senate Health Subcommittee held further hearings. Two former assistants to a Boston physician testified that he had given veterinary drugs to his patients, removing the bright orange labels warning "not for human use." He had assured them of having the manufacturer's approval to do so, but when they called the company, it expressed shock that the drug was being given to humans.

Another witness testified to falsifying records for her former husband, a physician and researcher. "I felt uncomfortable about being involved in testing, but I felt pressured to do it," she said.

An FDA official described a series of instances in which independent investigators for drug companies faked their test results. One called on the carpet for numerous inconsistencies in his data explained that he was a compulsive worker, to such a degree, in fact, that he had to take his paperwork home with him. "He said that the original records were lost in a rowboat accident. The investigator said he had taken the records with him in a boat on a lake, the boat tipped over, and the data went to the bottom in a metal box and was irretrievable." He then had to make up new records which, the FDA testified, were not based on fact. (35)

The 1980s have witnessed more cases of scientific fraud than ever before, and clinical trials have not been exempt from the overall deterioration.

In 1987 William K. Summers, M.D., a California psychiatrist who in 1986 had published (in the *New England Journal of Medicine*) a study of tetrahydroaminoacridine (THA, *Tacrine*) in Alzheimer's Disease, and who had claimed dramatic improvement of memory and functioning in these patients, was unable to provide crucial records documenting these patients' conditions. He argued that records which had been "...'rearranged, tampered with, or deleted,' were the responsibility of an assistant who was later fired." He admitted that randomization of patients was done arbitrarily by an office assistant, not by computer-generated random numbers. Although this cast substantial doubt on the validity of his results, the National Institute on Aging unaccountably decided to proceed with a large-scale trial. (36)

In 1988 Stephen Breuning, M.D., who had built a reputation as a leading authority on drug treatment of the mentally retarded, pled guilty in federal court to falsifying scientific data to obtain federal grants. (37)

In 1988 a New Jersey rheumatologist, Robert A. Fogari, M.D., pled guilty to four counts of falsifying, fabricating, and inventing data from 1977 to 1985 while conducting experimental drug studies for which he was paid $1.85 million by drug manufacturers. He had participated in at least eighteen studies. (38)

Fraud and falsification of data are seen, by spokesmen for American medicine, as regrettable aberrations in an otherwise bright picture of medical progress. James Wyngaarden, Director of the National Institutes of Health, which supports many clinical trials, stated in 1988: "that there should be a few cases per year of egregious dishonesty is regrettable, but I don't think it indicts the entire enterprise." (39)

But the argument can be made that the likelihood of fraud is a built-in feature of clinical trial procedure. The investigator, after all, is being paid sizable sums by the very manufacturer of the drug, and the financial temptation to perform dishonest trials is strong. While clinical investigation is not a prestigious area of medical activity, it can be lucrative. Many, like Robert Fogari, M.D., are known to gross more than $1 million annually from their testing programs. (40)

Americans who readily admit that politicians do favors for campaign contributors and that officials of the Defense Department throw contracts to suppliers with whom they later take salaried positions sometimes seem to feel that conflicts of interest are unknown in medicine. But physicians are, of course, subject to these same temptations. The would-be fraudulent clinical investigator, in fact, has strong inducements to follow the path of least resistance and little concern about possible punishment for his transgressions.

The probability of being caught is rather minimal, while the penalties for medical fraud are laughable.

Audits are labor-intensive and expensive and must be applied selectively. Hence, the vast majority of clinical trials are never audited by the FDA. (41)

And the likelihood of exposure by physicians performing the same study is equally infinitesimal. Trials are rarely replicated, and discrepencies can readily be presented as resulting from the methodological weaknesses and incongruities mentioned earlier.

The penalties for fraud are lenient to nonexistent. The FDA's powers in this area are limited:

> The regulatory system makes it extremely difficult and expensive for the FDA to disqualify from further research an investigator who does not go willingly. Because the burden of proof is on the FDA, investigators who are incompetent or dishonest may be able to ply their trade with impunity. (Martin F. Shapiro, M.D. and Robert P. Charrow, J.D., 1989)(42)

Most of the time the investigator is urged to "sin no more," and then *permitted to continue testing drugs as before.*

> Since the FDA, like any federal regulatory agency, has limited resources, it concentrates its disciplinary efforts on the most serious offenses identified. In other cases, it requires the investigators to indicate in writing what they have done to rectify the problems identified... until recently, formal assurances that they would not do it again were accepted by the FDA in lieu of sanctions from some investigators who had committed serious and deliberate offenses... Seventeen investigators (4%) who had repeatedly and deliberately violated regulations, and who had engaged in scientific misconduct according to our definition of the term, provided assurances to the FDA that they would not continue to do so in their future research, thereby avoiding disqualification. (Martin F. Shapiro, M.D. and Robert P. Charrow, J.D., 1989)(43)

Manufacturers have no particular reason to boycott M.D. investigators who obtain positive results by fabricating data:

> While pharmaceutical manufacturers may withhold funding from investigators who conduct studies poorly and may well seek out respected investigators, they are under no obligation to do so. (Martin F. Shapiro, M.D. and Robert P. Charrow, J.D., 1989)(44)

In fact, one may assume that manufacturers welcome the collaboration of investigators who, for a price, provide the data needed. Dale Console, M.D. described what the Squibb Company did in the 1950s when one of its investigators was caught cheating:

> I remember clearly an occasion when we were making preliminary studies of a drug that was being produced in very small quantities by a laboratory operation. We sent a highly placed authority enough of the drug to treat two patients and were somewhat puzzled by the fact that he sent us favorable data on three patients. When, shortly thereafter, he sent us laboratory data containing an item dated one day after the postmark on the letter, we blacklisted him. To put the incident in its proper context I must confess that blacklisting him consisted in taking his name out of the file of reliable investigators who could serve as adequate guides to important decisions. His card was transferred to another file that indicated that he could be used as a proof-mill when and if we should have need for one.
>
> There were proof mills that would deliver data at so much per head and in extreme cases we used them. There were drugs that were declared useless after clinical trial by experts that subsequently became marketable using the testimonials of less experienced physicians to prepare a New Drug Application. (Dale Console, M.D., 1969)(45)

This practice was not discontinued after passage of the Kefauver-Harris Amendment. When asked by a journalist in 1973 if investigators and drug companies ever collude to deceive the government, Alan Lisook replied: "There are companies who are not above hiring investigators who will give them the results they desire." (46)

A final point worth bearing in mind is that fraudulent conclusions from clinical trials continue to live on and influence future clinical decisions. A 1990 survey, by Mark P. Pfeifer, M.D. and Gwendolyn L. Snodgrass, of 82 studies published in professional journals between 1973 and 1983 and later retracted as invalid, found that they were cited 733 times in the specialized literature. "The 733 scientific citations were not the result of articles being too far along in the publishing process to be corrected when retractions were announced," they wrote. The articles of one researcher, John R. Darsee, M.D., of the Harvard Medical School, who had achieved national, even international, notoreity when his fraud was revealed, were still cited no less than 123 times after Darsee's retraction had been published. Pfeifer and Snodgrass attributed the longevity of fraudulent data to the fact that retractions were *not indexed*, even in the journals in which they were published; also, the format of the retraction was irregular: sometimes a letter to the editor, sometimes a full-page advertisement, sometimes a small notice in the back of the journal. (47)

Just as automobiles can be designed for safety, so scientific procedures can be made more or less susceptible to fraudulent manipulation. The controlled clinical trial, which despite its imposing name is a utopian but shaky intellectual edifice with many areas of methodologic uncertainty and many opportunities for the physician to cut corners, offers powerful temptations to researchers who find that the established protocol does not yield the data they want.

While no one maintains that every single clinical trial suffers from the vices and defects noted above, the fact that one quarter of all trials do not follow the established protocol and one quarter cannot furnish adequate data may well "indict the entire enterprise."

# VII. STATISTICAL ANALYSIS

The last stage of the trial is processing the data for "statistical significance."

The very real danger here is that the statistician will rely on the physician to make sense out of an often confused and muddy clinical picture, while the physician will place his hopes in the statistician:

> The clinician, forgetting the importance of his own contribution to the logic and data of the research, becomes mesmerized by what he does not understand: the statistical analysis. He assumes that the statistical computations will somehow validate the more basic activities, rectifying errors in observation and correcting distorted logic. The statistician, believing that problems in the basic logic and data have already been resolved, or are unresolvable, becomes oblivious to what he does not understand: the clinical background of the descriptive statistics. He accepts the data as presented, and he concentrates on the way he will fit them into his array of analytical statistical maneuvers.... What emerges is often an elaborately analyzed "statistically significant" collection of bad logic and bad data whose scientific deficiencies are not merely neglected but actually embellished and convoluted amid the mass of numbers and statistical tests. (Alvan Feinstein, M.D., 1977)(1)

The first contribution to the "collection of bad logic and bad data" is made by both parties during initial editing of the data. They will have been compiled in crude form during the trial, and must now be "tidied up":

> There is more error and bias unwittingly introduced into clinical trials at the data editing stage than from any other single factor in the procedure ... The bias introduced by the need to edit badly designed record cards goes a long way to explain some of the discrepancies between and within trials. (J.J.Grimshaw, 1970)(2)

A common procedure at the editing stage, especially in cancer trials, is simply to ignore patients who have dropped out of the study:

> Exclusion of patients because "they were lost to follow-up" or "they died too soon to be assessed" is common. Any patient who satisfies criteria for entry into a trial but who fails to return to clinic or dies soon after treatment is a nonresponder, and to label him or her otherwise borders on dishonesty. (Ian Tannock, M.D. and Kevin Murphy, M.D., 1983)(3)

Martin Shapiro, M.D. gives another example of editing malpractice:

> Let's take an experiment in which eighty people have a cancer, and half of them are going to be treated with an experimental drug, and the other half are going to receive a placebo. People are generally randomized between these two treatments. So of eighty subjects, forty are assigned to the experimental group. They will receive the drug. And the others are assigned to the control group. What then happens is that we see in the control group that six months later twenty of them are dead, shall we say, and twenty are alive. In the experimental group, twenty-nine are alive and eleven are dead. This is a statistically significant difference. This is publishable. If it's an important tumor, if it's a new development in the management of that disease,

it would undoubtedly be published in an important journal.

But let's take the same experiment and have the results come out a little differently. And I mean just a little differently. Instead of twenty-nine survivors out of forty, let's make it twenty-eight...[twenty-eight survivors out of forty is a result that could occur by chance more than five percent of the time]. Thus, this result does not achieve statistical significance...

The investigator looking at the findings, he might say, "Gosh, I really believe this treatment works, this is an important advance in the management of this disease. How unfortunate that we're just not quite at that level to be called statistically significant."

What's he to do? Well, a very normal response is to want to go back and look at the data and make sure that he didn't get it wrong, make sure that there isn't something there that doesn't reveal the truth as he knows it to be. And so he goes and looks, and he decides that one of these twelve cases of people who were treated who died was someone who perhaps didn't receive all of the medication, or perhaps didn't quite meet the criteria for entry into the study. And he decides that that person shouldn't have been in the experiment. And so he drops him from the experiment. And suddenly there are only eleven of thirty-nine who died. This is statistically significant again.

The unethical conduct would be not to report these kinds of manipulations of the data.

Now the perfectly ethical investigator would continue to collect data, expand his sample size. If the same trend remained it would reach statistical significance at some point. But that might take another year or two to do. This person might not have time or the patience to do that. (4)

It is quite obvious that the controlled clinical trial, with its general methodological fuzziness, will readily lend itself to this kind of trimming.

The above example illustrates an important distinction which physicians do not always comprehend — namely, the difference between statistical and clinical significance.

> The biostatistical malpractice committed with tests of "significance" has become a scandal, and the phrase, "statistical significance," has become such a malignant mental pathogen that major efforts to excise it will be undertaken. (Alvan Feinstein, M.D., 1977)(5)

In the first part of the above example a P value of .05 was attained, but this does not mean that the treatment was unambiguously responsible for the better recovery rate. Once in every twenty such trials a P value of .05 will be attained merely through the operation of chance. Thus this trial could have "statistical" significance without possessing any "clinical" significance.

By the same token, failure to attain a P value of .05 does not preclude a causal relationship between treatment and recovery. The statistician decides that the outcome "could" have been due to chance, but that does not mean it *was* necessarily due to chance. (6) The P value of .05 is arbitrary. A higher or lower one could have been chosen. (7) The treatment could well have "clinical significance," which would become clear if the test were repeated. The physician has only to increase his sample size. If the trend observed a sample of ten — i.e., the ratio of deaths to survivals — is still seen in a sample of fifty or one hundred, "clinical" significance gradually becomes "statistical" significance.

Or a different hypothesis could have been selected, one which would have been better supported by the data.

The physician cannot and should not be guided merely by statistical manipulations in evaluating the results of a trial. He has the right to introduce other elements in judging whether it is a success or a failure.

All the statistician can do is to make allowances for

assignable causes of variation and hence present the analysis in such a way that it will aid your decision. The responsibility for assigning *clinical* significance is yours and yours alone. Statisticians can do many things, but they cannot work miracles — that is your job. (J.J.Grimshaw, 1970)(8)

In any case, statisticians do not always agree on the meaning of the clinical data:

The best technique I know is never to have an even number of biostatisticians on any committee that has to make decisions. (Thomas C. Chalmers, M.D., 1971)(9)

# VIll. THE CLINICAL TRIAL: FOR OR AGAINST?

The preceding discussion has shown that the utopian ideal of the controlled clinical trial is rather far removed from the reality.

According to the ideal (especially when physicians are addressing non-medical audiences): (1) the procedure itself is "scientific," (2) practice is in accord with theory, (3) the clinical trial is the only reliable way to discover new therapeutic knowledge, and (4) its results have a marked impact on medical practice, inducing doctors to adopt or reject treatments as they are demonstrated effective or ineffective.

The reality (when physicians are addressing one another) is different: (1) the controlled clinical trial is not "scientific" in any sense of the word, (2) it is rarely, if ever, conducted as theory stipulates, (3) it is not the only way, and not even a very useful way, to discover new therapeutic knowledge, and (4) it does not affect physicians' prescribing habits as it is supposed to do.

Let us examine these four points in order and then return to the question of the true socio-economic significance of the clinical trial.

## The Clinical Trial is Not A Scientific Procedure

If the trial is to be considered "scientific," it must follow the rules of scientific method.

The four stages of scientific investigation, as described by the philosopher F.S.C.Northrop, consist of: (1) analysis of the problem, (2) description of its elements, (3) formulation of a hypothesis, and (4) testing the hypothesis under controlled conditions.

Of these stages the most interesting for our purposes is (2) — what Northrop calls the "natural history stage."

> As a rule, it involves not one method but three: namely, the method of observation, the method of description, and the method of classification ... The second stage of inquiry comes to an end when the facts designated by the analysis of the problem in the first stage are immediately apprehended by observation, expressed in terms of concepts with carefully denotative meanings by description, and systematized by classification. (1)

This stage of investigation cannot be ignored or slighted:

> If one proceeds immediately to the ... third stage of inquiry before one has passed through the natural history type of science ... appropriate to the second stage, the result is immature, half-baked, dogmatic, and for the most part worthless theory. (2)

But the clinical trial is an attempt to implement Northrop's stages (3) and (4) — the formulation and testing of a hypothesis (usually taking the form: Medicine A will be effective against Disease X) — without first doing justice to stage (2).

Hence the medical knowledge developed is often "immature, half-baked, dogmatic, and for the most part worthless." This goes far to explain why the clinical trial today is in a state of crisis.

The irremediable defect of these trials is inability to cope with the heterogeneity of the subject matter. Before formulating hypotheses and attempting to test them on patients, physicians must first observe, describe, and classify the subject-matter of the investigation. But, as we saw in Chapters II and III, the object of the clinical trial — the "disease entity," the "homogeneous sample" — cannot be "observed, described, and classified" other than in terms of the common features of a group of disparate individuals. The object of the clinical trial is an abstraction which has no actual existence:

> Does science consist of precise identification, accurate prediction, and valid specification, or does it consist of statistical correlations? Very often it consists of both, but unless we have the identifications and specifications, how good are the correlations? I maintain that at the moment we rely on correlations without any real attempt to achieve identification and specifications. (Alvan Feinstein, M.D., 1971)(3)

The clinical trial is an experiment performed on an unreal, unknown, mysterious entity — an assembly of sick people who have some features in common. Its results cannot be extrapolated to any larger population, and the information cannot be reliably duplicated.

What is worse, the results of the trial cannot even be extrapolated to the individual patient, who (not some faceless member of a "homogeneous group") is still the object of medical ministration.

> The controlled trial ... does not tell the doctor what he wants to know. It may be so constituted as to show without any doubt that treatment A is on the average better than treatment B. On the other hand, that result does not answer the practising doctor's question what is the most likely outcome when this drug is given to a particular patient. Is there indeed any way of answering that? (A.B.Hill, 1966)(4)

> Medical schools teach you to memorize what you don't understand and to solve problems by answering multiple-choice questions. Well, patients are not multiple choices ... Patients recognize their own uniqueness, even if we do not. (Lawrence L. Weed, M.D., 1974)(5)

> What is archaic in clinical medicine today is ... the idea that the complex natural phenomena occurring in diseased people can be adequately classified by a

taxonomy devoted only to disease... The clinician knows all these ... distinctly clinical features that are his harbingers of prognosis and determinants of therapy. But he cannot express them specifically or consistently. Medical taxonomy has given him classifications for the host and for the disease, but not for the illness of the patient who is the diseased host. (Alvan Feinstein, M.D., 1976)(6)

The patient must not be viewed as merely one subject in a population but rather as a unique individual who may or may not benefit from such treatment. (Howard S. Friedman, M.D., 1986)(7)

We test a therapeutic manoeuvre on a group of like subjects and use the results to predict the response of similar subjects in the future. But like subjects do not exist, and the groups and subgroups of patients studied in clinical trials are similar only with respect to a very few parameters. This type of experimentation ... may lead us to believe that all we have to do to optimize patient care is to apply these generalizations. Facts generated in this way, unfortunately, are only true of large groups and degenerate again into uncertainties when applied to individuals. Clinical problems cannot be solved by best fitting the patient to a group about which general truths are known while ignoring variables which have not received sympathetic study. (William J. MacKillop, M.D. and Pauline A. Johnston, 1986)(8)

Of course the juggernaut rolls on because the FDA regulations so specify and because clinical trials have several very powerful constituencies, but this procedure is in no sense scientific and should not be braced up and fortified by the full panoply and majesty of the law.

## Practice Differs from Theory

Not only is the clinical trial theoretically deficient, its practice is far removed from even the degenerated ideal — at best a trade-off between scientific and economic constraints:

Having been associated with numerous clinical trials, we cannot recall any that have been entirely satisfactory. All have entailed some compromise short of the ideal. (T.B.Binns, M.D., 1964)(9)

The perfect trial has never been achieved. Most trials suffer from defects of one sort or another, such as the need to administer agents other than the one in question (because of ethically required fail-safe clauses), the breaking of the double-blind because of the production of side effects by the active agent, differences in baseline variables in treatment groups in the study, and the occurrence of drop-outs... The more practical-minded individual settles for a good deal less than the ideal, realizing that the latter is not attainable. (Louis Lasagna, M.D., 1971)(10)

The design and administration of clinical trials are important interrelated aspects that require many compromises between the art of the possible and the theoretical ideal. (James E. Grizzle, Ph.D., 1982)(11)

Donald Fredrickson, M.D., Director of the National Institutes of Health, observed in 1977 that of 31,000 clinical trials conducted during the previous decade in the field of gastroenterology, only 1% had been randomized; closer scrutiny of a sample of 100 led to the conclusion that *none* satisfied the requirements for a convincing trial. (12)

Inability to attain the ideal is often blamed, by protagonists of the controlled clinical trial, on insufficiency of natural and human resources: there are just too few patients and physicians, (they maintain), there is too little money or time, to perform the study they would prefer to see done.

That is an error. The procedure is defective in its root and cannot be corrected by investing more money, time, manpower, or womanpower. The greater the volume of resources invested, the more glaringly the inherent vice of the procedure — its incapacity to deal with patient heterogeneity — is exposed to view.

## It is Not the Best Way to Discover New Therapeutic Knowledge

Its theoretical insufficiency and the insuperable obstacles to its practical implementation render the clinical trial an inadequate technique for discovering new therapeutic knowledge.

Soviet-American arms-control negotiations have been described as achieving success when they are no longer needed. The same can be said about the clinical trial. If it yields valuable data, this merely demonstrates that it was never needed in the first place, as the same information could have been obtained in better ways. True therapeutic advances become evident without resort to the clinical trial, and this procedure is used largely to make laborious distinctions among nearly identical forms of treatment:

> A great deal too much has been made of the controlled trial of remedies, for the greatest advances in therapy have come without them, and, in a large number of cases — for instance, malaria, meningococcal meningitis, pneumonia, diabetes, pernicious anemia, and myxedema — there are clear clinical or laboratory tests which will rapidly tell whether the treatment is effective ... a controlled clinical trial is quite often the wrong way to assess the value of a medical or surgical treatment. (Robert Platt, M.D., 1963)(13)

> Some therapies are so clearly beneficial, such as the use of penicillin for pneumococcal pneumonia or subacute bacterial endocarditis, that their efficacy is readily apparent. (Howard S. Friedman, M.D., 1986)(14)

But many extoll the clinical trial precisely for its supposed ability to make incremental contributions to the accumulation of medical knowledge:

Large improvements in clinical medicine make themselves known. It is the small improvements that will be missed without careful, controlled work. (Byron Browne, Jr., Ph.D., 1980)(15)

But how effective is the controlled clinical trial in yielding these "small improvements"?

Discussion of this issue is complicated by unwillingness of the parties to recognize that they are often engaged in a waste of their own time and other people's money (frequently, that of the taxpayer). The amounts involved are sizable. Some major projects of recent decades have been: the Coronary Drug Project ($41,336,083), the Hypertension Detection and Follow-Up Program (over $60,000,000), the Multiple Risk Factor Intervention Trial ($115,769,176), and the Coronary Primary Prevention Trial ($142,864,000). These are only a small part of the 8-10,000 trials ongoing in any given year. (16)

Why should the biomedical community criticize an undertaking which brings it so many tangible benefits?

Even so, the clinical trial literature is enlightening.

In the first place, it is generally admitted that trials all too often reach inconclusive or contradictory results.

A number of field trials in our day that have dealt with the value of anticoagulants or the effects of various drugs and diets upon atherosclerosis can be kindly said to have "ended in equivocation." They invite the mental image of a white-coated figure endlessly and unsuccessfully pursuing Truth across the Elysian Fields. It is not that we must always have a positive result or that we abhor the thought of a negative. It is the drawing of *neither* that is so unsettling. (Donald Fredrickson, M.D., 1968)(17)

I unequivocally believe that antidepressants are effective but also unequivocally believe that it is possible to pick an experimental population where the performance of the drug will be difficult to demonstrate. That is how I interpret the trials in the literature. There are positive trials, and there are negative trials which are simply not explainable by population size. They are explainable, I suppose, in terms of the disease process or sloppiness in defining depression, or a variety of things I know little about... In analgesics you have the same problem. I do not doubt that aspirin is an effective analgesic. I have also run a good many trials where it has not been possible to distinguish a placebo. (Louis Lasagna, M.D., 1971)(18)

Two frequent causes of these contradictory results are either methodologic, when trials incorporate design errors that lead to overt bias; or statistical, when too few patients are enrolled in a trial to provide reasonable assurance that a meaningful therapeutic difference would not be missed. A third source of conflicting trial results is the variation in trial designs employed by investigators studying the identical disease and therapy. The variation occurs because the randomized clinical trial is a paradigm with recognized components but without specific rules for how the components are to be defined or applied. (Ralph I. Horwitz, M.D., 1987)(19)

In 1982 two papers on the use of sodium nitroprusside for patients with acute myocardial infarction — one concluding that it reduced mortality and the other finding identical mortality rates in the treatment and control groups — appeared in the same issue of the peer-reviewed *New England Journal of Medicine.* (20)

The Hypertension Detection and Follow-Up Program (cost $60 million) and the Multiple Risk Factor Intervention Trial (cost $115 million), investigating the relationship between high blood pressure and heart disease, were ultimately inconclusive:

Their results have been questioned, and their application to therapeutic issues remains controversial. Overall, the Hypertension Detection and Follow-Up Program demonstrated a favorable outcome for the experimental group. However, analysis of subgroups did not contain sufficient patients for small differences in mortality to reach statistical significance, and a threshold at which mild hypertension should be treated could not be identified. The Multiple Risk Factor Intervention Trial produced confusing results. Mortality rates were less than expected on the basis of previous population studies, but the differences in mortality between the experimental and control groups were small and not statistically significant.

Interpretations of the results of these trials have been disputed because of the treatment received by the control groups. The control groups were referred to regular medical care sources in the community. Ethics were a central issue in this strategy. The Hypertension Detection and Follow-Up Program stated: "it is unethical not to recommend medical evaluation to probable or suspect hypertensives." In the Multiple Risk Factor Intervention Trial design, "the basic argument for this approach was ethical."

However, this strategy produced difficulties in the scientific evaluation of the results. Administrative factors and access to care differed for the experimental group, and these factors may have been important in the medical outcomes. The community sources did not adopt a no-treatment approach. *Many members of the control group were given the same treatment that was being investigated in the experimental group.* [added] Comparisons of the experimental and control groups suggested that many factors other than the intervention under study influenced the outcomes, but the design of the trials precluded the removal of these factors in the analyses of the outcomes. (Stephen T. Miller, M.D. and C. Perry, Ph.D., 1984)(21)

One could have hoped that a study costing taxpayers $115 million would avoid such an elementary blunder as allowing both test and control groups to receive the same treatment!

The *British Medical Journal* in 1987 lamented the "dispiritingly large number of current treatments for which uncertainty about efficiency and safety remains" and ascribed this to "the equivocal results of many small trials." (22)

What the doctor would like to know is how [a new drug] stacks up against the others. In what way is it better or worse — more effective and safer? Does it have a different spectrum of toxicity or of clinical disorder? Are certain groups of patients going to respond well? It is here where we are often lacking information, and this is not just the fault of the industry. *It is the fault of all of us and of the present technology.* [added]... We may be able to tease out which patients respond better to drug A than to drug B, and which respond with toxicity to drug A rather than to drug B... [but] if we are ever going to have improved therapeutics, we have to focus more clearly on relative efficacy and safety. We now act as if we are terribly wise about all this. Each physician juggles those P values for good and evil that seem to be available with precision. But the P values are not available with precision. Sometimes they are not available at all. We will not be in good shape until we seriously think about this problem and work hard at collecting data. (Louis Lasagna, M.D., 1971)(23)

A relatively small fraction of medical practice is devoted to life-saving or dramatic cures; most of it concerns efforts to relieve discomfort and dysfunction, and much of it can be expected to achieve small improvements at best. The experimental evidence on which to judge the effectiveness of most such cures is, unfortunately, poor. Nevertheless, physicians must make decisions ... The moral would appear to be: let's improve our capacity to improve health care ... Florence Nightingale, after returning from the Crimean War where she was appalled by the infections she saw in hospitalized soldiers, begged for better data on the outcomes of medical care. Today we have just begun to respond to the request. (John Bunker, M.D., 1980)(24)

But what if the trial really does seem to show slight benefit from a new therapy, meaning that a very large sample has been used. Does this not justify the procedure?

The answer, unfortunately, is "no," and the reason is to be found in yet another "therapeutic paradox":

> The larger the size of the sample required to establish the efficacy of a therapy, the smaller will be the probability of it benefiting a given person. The corollary of this logical relation is that the larger the size needed to show benefit, the greater will be the number who would receive the treatment without apparent benefit, yet remain exposed to the risks and side effects that it might produce. (Howard S. Friedman, M.D., 1986)(25)

Small but statistically significant improvements in treatment are accompanied by large risks of adverse reactions:

> then the pain and suffering therapy causes become the paramount consideration. Sometimes, the side effects are subtle, such as the mild depression and reduced exercise tolerance that may occur with beta-blockers administered following an acute myocardial infarction. *Often, as in the case of these drugs, symptoms of the drug are attributed to the event for which the drug has been prescribed and not recognized until after the medicine has been discontinued.* [added] For other treatments, the physical and psychological trauma is conspicuously apparent, such as when patients are subjected to a prophylactic coronary bypass operation, or perhaps coronary angioplasty, because of the statistical advantages determined by randomized clinical trials.

(Howard S. Friedman, M.D., 1986)(26)

An example of such an effort, in early 1990, was the decision by researchers at Oxford University to seek statistical significance by combining the results of fourteen inconclusive trials on the relationship between lowered blood pressure and the risk of heart attack. They claimed that lumping all 37,000 patients together into one monster group yielded "solid" evidence that reducing blood pressure lowers the risk of heart disease. Richard Peto, M.D., the project leader, called this "meta-analysis" a scientific breakthrough. Instead of attempting to control for every variable, he argued, data collection must be stripped to the essentials: Which patient is taking which drug, and is he or she getting better? While critics argued that Peto was comparing apples and oranges, he maintained that, with a large enough population, differences in age, sex, and other factors would average out. (27)

This is an illegitimate procedure for the reasons already given. If such a large sample is needed to demonstrate tiny differences between treating and not treating, most sample members will not benefit from treatment, while all are exposed to the medicine's side effects. The overall result is a deterioration in patient health.

The side effects are the joker in the deck.

The typical antihypertensive drug often does more harm than the disease it is designed to treat.

Let us look at spironolactone (*Aldactone*, G.D. Searle), a diuretic used as one of the main antihypertensive drugs.

This substance first made history in 1976 when the manufacturer admitted never having communicated to the FDA the results of tests showing it to cause cancer. Malignant tumors — which the regulations define as "alarming findings" — had been excised from the test rats; some listed as dead were later recorded as alive, then dead again, then resurrected once or even twice more. (28) Sales of *Aldactone* in 1974 had attained $87 million. (29) An FDA task-force was dispatched to Searle's Illinois plant, and its report concluded:

At the heart of FDA'a regulatory process is its ability to rely upon the integrity of the basic safety data submitted by sponsors of regulated products. Our investigation clearly demonstrates that, in the G.D.Searle Company, we have no basis for such reliance now. We have uncovered serious deficiencies in Searle's operations and practices which undermine the basis for reliance on Searle integrity in conducting high-quality animal research to accurately determine or characterize the toxic potential of its products. Searle made a number of deliberate decisions which seemingly were calculated to minimize the chances of discovering toxicity and/or to allay FDA concern. (30)

Even so, *Aldactone* is still today prescribed three million times a year for hypertension despite a prominent warning in the *Physicians' Desk Reference*:

Spironolactone has been shown to be a tumorigen in chronic toxicity studies in rats ... Unnecessary use of this drug should be avoided. (31)

And future participants in "meta-analytic" studies of antihypertensive drug therapy would do well first to read carefully all the "adverse reactions" attributed to *Aldactone*:

Gynecomastia [swelling of the breasts in men] is observed not infrequently. A few cases of agranulocytosis [change in the composition of the blood] have been reported ... Other adverse reactions that have been reported in association with *Aldactone* are: gastrointestinal symptoms including cramping and diarrhea, drowsiness, lethargy, headache, maculopapular or erythematous cutaneous eruptions, urticaria, mental confusion, drug fever, ataxia [irregular jerky muscular movements], inability to achieve or maintain erection, irregular menses or amenorrhoea, postmenopausal bleeding, hirsutism, deepening of the voice, gastric bleeding, ulceration, gastritis, and vomiting. Carcinoma of the breast has been reported in patients taking spironolactone, but a cause and effect relationship has not been established. (32)

Another excessively popular drug in recent decades has been clofibrate (*Atromid*, Ayerst Laboratories), a leading cholesterol-reducing agent. The Coronary Drug Project in the late 1960s found not only that cholesterol was not reduced at all, or just barely, but that this substance was *ineffective* in treating patients with myocardial infarction. (33) The OTA *Background Paper* notes:

> All completed randomized clinical trials of lipid intervention for atherosclerotic cardiovascular disease have shown no convincing evidence for disease retardation, arrest, or reversal associated with plasma cholesterol reduction; albeit in no trial has cholesterol reduction been marked, and in many it has been minuscule. (34)

But "adverse reactions" from *Atromid* occupy a whole column in the *Physicians' Desk Reference*: "cardiovascular" (increased or decreased angina, arrhythmias, phlebitis), "dermatologic" (rashes, pruritus, baldness, allergic reactions), "gastrointestinal" (nausea, diarrhea, vomiting, bloating, flatulence, stomatitis, gastritis, swollen liver, abnormal liver function, gallstones), "genitourinary" (impotence and decreased libido, kidney dysfunction), "hematologic" (anemia and other blood disorders), "musculoskeletel" (cramps, "flu-like" symptoms, arthralgia), "neurologic" (fatigue, weakness, drowsiness, dizziness, headache), "miscellaneous" (weight gain and bulimia).

Reported adverse reactions whose direct relationship with the drug have not been established are: peptic ulcer, gastrointestinal hemorrhage, rheumatoid arthritis, tremors, increased perspiration, systemic lupus erythematosus, blurred vision, gynecomastia, and thrombocytopenic purpura. (35)

One may assume that such a "direct relationship" will be established in time. What is more, a World Health Organization study found "a statistically significant 36% higher mortality due to noncardiovascular causes in the *Atromid*-treated group than in a comparable placebo-treated group. Half of this difference was due to malignancy." (36) Some of the deaths in the WHO study were due to the complications of gall-bladder operations. (37) Today *Atromid* is still prescribed 300-400,000 times a year in the United States.

If an individual with mild hypertension or elevated cholesterol should take *Atromid* or *Aldactone*, he will get no clinical benefit at all from the first, and a modest lowering of the blood pressure (through increased urination) from the second. From both, however, he (or she) may get tumors, other malignancies, gallstones, gall-bladder inflammation, pancreatitis, and all the rest of the wearisome catalogue of "adverse reactions" which seemingly accompanies every new drug introduced to the market.

These reactions have never been adequately factored into therapeutic equations. A General Accounting Office report in 1973 found that drug companies were simply concealing from the FDA data on side effects of drugs undergoing clinical trials. The time lag was as long as nineteen months. The report also complained that follow-up examinations of persons receiving experimental drugs were not always undertaken, even when these drugs were later found to cause cancer in animals. (38)

A notorious instance was the reluctance of Merrell Laboratories in 1971 to examine the vision of patients testing a drug later found to cause cataracts in animals; a year after the FDA had made the request, less than half the patients had been so examined. (39)

In 1985 the Eli Lilly Co. pled guilty to criminal charges for failure to report several dozen deaths and non-fatal cases of liver and kidney failure in British patients receiving its new anti-arthritis drug, *Oraflex*, in a trial. The Lilly Co. had been kept regularly informed by telex of all adverse reactions, but by April, 1982, when *Oraflex* was approved for release in the United States, these had not yet been reported to the FDA. In the following fourteen weeks U.S. sales of *Oraflex* totaled $14 million. By August, when it was withdrawn, there had been

62 deaths in England and another eleven in the United States, and the eventual death toll was 120 in the two countries, with 200 additional instances of non-fatal liver and kidney failure. The Lilly vice-president in charge of *Oraflex* later stated in court that he had not reported the deaths because none of them "was unexpected in relation to this class of chemical agent." But he pled guilty to fifteen misdemeanor counts, was fined $15,000, and went on to become research director of a major British pharmaceutical manufacturer. (40)

There is no reason to assume that these practices have ceased.

And even when adverse reactions are reported, they are not properly incorporated into the evaluation of the drug. As the OTA *Background Paper* notes: "Adverse effects ... are usually analyzed separately from indications of effectiveness in comparing therapies." (41) A Finnish researcher has suggested that adverse reactions and beneficial effects should be expressed using the same scale, as in cost-effectiveness analyses, but *this is not being done.*

In 1990 the General Accounting Office reported that over half the drugs approved as "safe" by the Food and Drug Administration between 1976 and 1985 caused such serious side effects as to require relabelling of the drug or its withdrawal from the market. These side effects were described as "common" and resulted in hospitalization, permanent disability, and even death. A member of the House of Representatives commented: "This is an important reminder that FDA approval does not guarantee that approved drugs are completely safe." (43)

What, then, does "safety" testing mean if one drug in two passing this test is later found to cause hospitalization, permanent disability, and/or death?

We may assume that our knowledge of adverse reactions is still rudimentary. As already noted, the information is not readily released by the manufacturers. Misrepresentation and concealment of data are encountered very commonly.

Even so, medical authorities in the early 1970s viewed adverse reactions to drugs as wholly or partly responsible for the deaths of between 0.5% and 1.5% of hospital patients. (44) A 1981 survey raised this figure. Based on 815 admissions to a university hospital and relying, in the authors' view, on "conservative criteria," Knight Steel, M.D. and coworkers found that in 2% of hospital admissions the "iatrogenic illness was believed to contribute to the death of the patient." (45)

There are 35,000,000 hospital admissions in the U.S. every year. If iatrogenic illness contributes to the patient's death in 2% of cases, 700,000 deaths per year in the United States (out of an overall mortality of two million) may be attributable, in whole or in part, to drug reactions.

Furthermore, adverse reactions often lead to "iatrogenic disease" and predispose the individual to a later chronic disease. (46) In 1987 almost 13% of the American population, 31 million people, suffered from one or another chronic disease, making it the country's major health problem. (47)

This high level of adverse reactions and, we may assume, the ensuing high incidence of iatrogenic and chronic disease, are due in large part to the fact that the United States is the most overmedicated society in the world, as confirmed by a 1977 World Health Organization study. (48)

> We cannot justify the treatment of minor illnesses with drugs which, in and of themselves, do more harm than the diseases they are presumably treating. (Leighton Cluff, M.D., 1971)(49)

Often enough, adverse reactions are not spotted against the overall background of the disease but are attributed to the event for which the drug has been prescribed. Or, as noted in 1977 by the Director of the National Institutes of Health:

> One of the most important lessons that trials and other epidemiologic studies have taught us in recent years is that adverse effects of drugs and other treatments may not be responses unique to the drug under study but may instead manifest themselves as an increased

incidence of a disorder that already occurs in the absence of the treatment. (Donald S. Fredrickson, M.D., 1977)(50)

Finally, the fabrication of new drug molecules has certainly given rise to whole new classes of adverse reactions of which we as yet know nothing, which are unpredictable and undiscoverable until it is too late. What Harry Dowling, M.D., stated in 1968 about congenital deformities from thalidomide is undoubtedly applicable today to new varieties of side effects:

> The thalidomide episode opens for us a Pandora's box of congenital deformities produced by drugs; yet we know so little about how and when they occur, what chemical configurations cause them, and how congenital deformities in animals relate to congenital deformities in man. We are still in a state of stunned bewilderment at the enormity of the problem. Sometimes it seems that we are doing little more at this stage than walk around in circles looking for the best animals to use for testing purposes. (Harry Dowling, M.D., 1968)(51)

When and if the true incidence of adverse reactions from the quantities of drugs consumed in our overmedicated society ever becomes known (how many other rats have had their tumors excised and been returned to the study?), we will have a real understanding of the meaning of drug "safety."

> Unless the scientific method of both innovative and conventional clinical therapy are made more sensible and reproducible, the widespread distribution of modern therapeutic agents may provoke iatrogenic tragedies worse, individually and collectively, than any already known in medical history. (Alvan Feinstein, M.D., 1976)(52)

## Clinical Trial Results Do Not Affect Prescribing Patterns

Thomas C. Chalmers, M.D. studied physicians' practice in the 1950s and 1960s and found it often at odds with the results of clinical trials. (53)

Patrick McGrady came to the same conclusion in a 1982 survey of family practitioners. (54)

According to the 1983 OTA *Background Paper,* "Most authors conclude that the impact of RCTs on medical practice has been less than optimal or that their impact is exceedingly slow to develop." (55)

The *British Medical Journal* editorialized in 1987 that clinical trials have "little immediate impact" because of their equivocal results. (56)

Participants in the Lugano Conference gave a variety of answers to the question: "Why do messages from CCTs filter into clinical medicine so slowly?" Ninety-five percent ascribed it to physicians' determination to rely exclusively on their own "personal experience." Eighty-four percent said that "medical journals distort the truth by favoring CCTs with positive results." Eighty-seven percent held that "prescribers should be educated in trials methodology so that they can base their decisions on their own assessment of published CCTs rather than rely on the possibly biased opinion of others." (57)

Practising physicians "do not know about published negative CCTs" because: "they rarely read medical journals" (75%), "sales representatives, their main source of information, rarely refer to negative CCTs" (93%), "negative CCTs are rarely abstracted in medical news magazines" (88%), and, finally, "they ignore them, since most negative CCTs are undersized and uninterpretable" (39%).

For whatever reason, physicians continue to prescribe medicines demonstrated ineffective by controlled clinical trials. And they sometimes reject a new treatment even when shown to be effective by this method.

A prominent Danish physician and gastroenterologist, chairman of his country's Medical Research Council, found in

1977 that trials of anticholinergic drugs for treatment of peptic ulcer, extending over thirteen years, had all shown them to be valueless in this condition. And yet the number of textbook recommendations of these substances for treating ulcers was steadily on the rise. (58) Today, in 1990, the anticholinergic drug, hexocyclium methylsulfate (*Tral*), for treating peptic ulcer is still on the market. (59)

Pentaerythritol tetranitrate (*Peritrate, Pentritol*) was shown by two double-blind studies in the late 1950s to be probably ineffective in coronary artery disease, and yet, as a physician observed in 1972, "the most widely prescribed coronary vasodilator today is still the one that is probably ineffective." (60) Today several types of pentaerythritol tetranitrate are still prescribed in this condition.

When clofibrate was shown to have no value in preventing recurrence of myocardial infarction in 1975, it was being prescribed 2,200,000 times a year; in 1980 it was still being prescribed 350,000 times per year. (61) A survey of cardiologists between 1979 and 1981 — ten to twelve years after the conclusions of the Coronary Disease Project had been published — found that 73% of those with "no" knowledge of the Project, 55% of those with "some" knowledge of the Project, and an astonishing 45.5% of those professing "full" knowledge of the Project, were nonetheless prescribing clofibrate. (62)

It will be recalled that the chief "adverse reaction" associated with this drug is a 36% higher overall mortality. (63)

Decades after five controlled studies at the University of Chicago and elsewhere from 1952 to 1955 had shown diethylstilbestrol (DES, stilbestrol) to be without benefit in preventing spontaneous abortion, physicians were still prescribing it to pregnant women for this purpose. As many as six million women may have taken it. (64) Even in 1958-1960 Thomas C. Chalmers, M.D. found only that "most" (not "all") textbooks of obstetrics were advising against this use of the drug. (65) Then a famous article in 1971 demonstrated a connection between stilbestrol therapy during pregnancy and cervical cancer in the *daughters* of these women, also genital and other abnormalities in their sons. (66) But in 1977 it was still being used in 1-2% of pregnancies in the United States — from 32,000 to 64,000 women — causing 582 to 1164 infants to be born every year with heart defects. (67)

In 1989 a thirteen-year-old Maryland girl, whose paternal *grandmother* had taken stilbestrol while pregnant, died of the same distinctive clear-cell adenocarcinoma of the vagina that has already occurred in several hundred "DES daughters." (68)

Bed rest for hepatitis was first advocated in 1945, then shown by a clinical trial in 1955 to be ineffective. But a 1973 survey of university hospitals found that physicians were still prescribing strict bed rest for 50% of their patients; in community hospitals the figure was 70%. (69)

The bland or "sippy" diet for peptic ulcer was first used in the late nineteenth century. It was then shown to be ineffective by eight published trials, but these took 37 years to be performed; and a 1973 survey of university and community hospitals found that 35 of 38 physicians were prescribing the bland or "sippy" diet for ulcer patients. (70)

The oral anti-diabetic drugs were introduced in 1954, and in 1970 the University Group Diabetes Program (costing $7.3 million) announced that these patients had proportionately more deaths from heart disease than those who controlled diabetes through diet or diet plus insulin. (71) The drugs, especially tolbutamide (*Orinase*, Upjohn) and chlorpropamide (*Diabinase*, Pfizer), continued to be administered to 1.5 million Americans in the mid-1970s, despite estimates that they were killing 10,000-15,000 diabetics each year. (72)

The findings of the UGDP were fought long and bitterly by diabetes specialists and the manufacturers, who presumably supported their patients' preference for a pill that could be swallowed rather than insulin which must be injected. In 1982, twelve years after the UGDP results had been published, they were still not mentioned on the package inserts for *Orinase* and *Diabinase*, which Thomas C. Chalmers, M.D. called "a real black mark on the Food and Drug Administration." (73)

The reason may be that in the early 1980s almost nine million prescriptions for oral antidiabetic drugs were being sold in the United States each year, including 1,400,000 for *Orinase* and 4,470,000 for *Diabinase.*

Not only are bad medicines not abandoned by physicians after adverse findings in controlled clinical trials, good medicines are not necessarily accepted. Abram Hoffer, M.D. has called attention to the nicotinic acid treatment for schizophrenia developed by him in 1952 and demonstrated effective by three double-blind controlled studies with follow-ups for as long as fourteen years. His ten-year cure rate is claimed to be 75%, compared to 35% in a comparison control group. (74) Today, almost forty years later, this therapy is still not accepted.

Finally, physicians may, and do, use drugs in ways which have never been justified by any controlled clinical trial. (75)

Once the regulatory body has agreed that these things are O.K., then the drug is marketed. Let's say the company markets it as a diuretic. There are all sorts of areas now in which it can be misused. The doctor may misdiagnose the illness the patient has and use the drug inappropriately. He may start using it and find that it is good for migraine or he thinks that it is. He starts using it for migraine or perhaps for lowering blood pressure or for something else which wasn't originally thought of as being the right purpose of the drug. (Owen L. Wade, M.D, 1971)(76)

In the light of these cases it would be difficult to maintain that clinical trials have a marked impact on medical practice.

## Loss of the Physician's Ability to Observe. Dehumanization

We stated in Chapter VI that "blinding" is a startling departure from the traditional ideal of the physician as observer. To the extent that the blinded clinical trial isolates physician from patient and makes him a less good observer, it contributes to the general deterioration of physician-patient relations in late twentieth-century medicine.

One thing fundamentally wrong is the design of the typical experiment using human subjects. All too often such experiments are set up in a manner that almost guarantees emotional distance and alienation between the experimenter and his subjects. It is not unusual for many contemporary researchers to have no personal knowledge of the identity of the participants in their own experiments, which are carried out via intermediaries. All too often scientific objectivity is distorted to include callousness and lack of concern for the human aspects of research. (Richard Restak, M.D., 1975)(77)

Austin Hill had hoped that the clinical trial would improve the physician's powers of observation:

Far from weakening the need for the skilled observer, the controlled trial should increase the demands. It most certainly must do so if part of the protocol of a trial is the attempt to identify features in the patient that favor or disfavor response to a specific treatment. That will call for a prepared and percipient mind. (Austin B. Hill, 1966)(78)

The evidence indicates that the opposite has occurred. A 1979 survey of clinical trials concluded that since 1947 reliance on laboratory tests had increased, while diagnosis from clinical signs and symptoms had declined significantly. "Similarly, the frequency with which the social, occupational, or emotional status of subjects has been reported has diminished with time." (79)

Some might maintain that the physician who is completely aloof from his patients is the most "scientific," but this would be a serious error. As long as the scientific elements of diagnosis remain as imperfect as they are today, as long as the patient's status cannot be described in objective numerical terms, the physician's ability to observe his patient, to sense intuitively those elements of his illness or wellness which cannot be quantified, will remain an important, even an essential, component of diagnosis and a vital necessity for successful treatment:

> Can we identify the individual patient for whom one or the other of the treatments is the right answer? Clearly that is what we want to do, and present-day investigators ought to give far more attention to the problem. There are very few signs that they are doing so. There are several ways in which this problem might be tackled. First we might take note of considerably more characteristics that delineate the patient — whether measurable features or observations of qualities. At the conclusion of the trial we should be able to see which, if any, of these characteristics had been associated with a favorable response to a specific treatment. Thus we might learn to specify the traits of the patient that are required for success ... The trouble is that with many diseases and many treatments we are too ignorant to know where even to look. (A.B.Hill, 1966)(80)

The "aloof" or "objective," meaning "dehumanized," physician is incapable of really observing, i.e., of really knowing, the patient before him (or her). The physician's obligation to observe carefully and correctly has not been superseded by all the methodologic subtleties of the clinical trial.

Dehumanization is carried to extreme lengths as physicians become more alienated from their patients and also more confident of the results of controlled clinical trials. Therapeutics is mistakenly viewed as a balancing of precisely delineated, and highly abstract, risks and benefits:

> Drug therapy today has become as precise as the surgeon's knife, and we in the profession have to remember that. (A.B.Taylor, M.D., 1972)(81)

> If I never hear *primum nil nocere* again it will be too soon. This philosophy is totally irrelevant in 1970. What do you mean, *first don't do any harm*? First do some good. What you are trying to do with these powerful

chemicals is to juggle the possibilities for good against the possibilities for evil... One could argue that the FDA ought to send "Dear Doctor" letters out when a new form of efficacy or usefulness comes out and not restrict itself to the more dramatic pronouncements on toxicity. If you are going to tell doctors about the risks of thromboembolism, you should also tell them about the risks of not using oral contraceptives ... (Louis Lasagna, M.D., 1971)(82)

This, in part, explains why physicians are willing to run risks with their patients — or, in any case, with other physicians' patients — and even  sacrifice them for the "good of society."

Benefit, in my view, must be considered not only in the light of amelioration of human disease, but also in the light of insights gained into biochemical or biophysical problems. The introduction of a novel compound in man rarely benefits only the disease for which it was introduced, but benefits all science and ultimately other diseases as well. (Roger Palmer, M.D., 1972)(83)

I would like to point out that there is no question but that we are all interested in the patient's protection. Patient protection, however, runs along two lines just like sin: omission and commission. It is very easy to see that if you put restrictions on a drug that produces toxicity you will thereby protect the patient. It is not so easy to see the harm done to a patient if you put restrictions on a drug which will be useful even though in the long run it may be toxic. Obviously, the efficacy must outweigh the toxicity, but the former will never be known if evaluation is stopped prematurely because of the overwhelming concern about toxicity. We need to be very careful that we don't make the latter type of error. (Daniel L. Azarnoff, M.D., 1972)(84)

In 1973 a Swedish medical professor and winner of the Nobel Prize in medicine urged that drugs be tested less on animals and more on people, to accelerate their introduction into practice. As it is, Ulf von Euler opined, new drugs are being delayed by "hyper-cautious" authorities out of fear of side effects:

> Since it is virtually impossible to foresee all actions of a drug, tragic events can never be excluded. In my opinion the community should take responsibility in such unhappy circumstances, just as it does in catastrophes of other kinds, when victims are compensated. (85)

Twenty-two notorious examples of the sacrificing of patients for the supposed good of society, involving death, serious illness, and unnecessary and dangerous operations, were described in 1966 by Henry K. Beecher, M.D., professor at the Harvard Medical School.

Ordinary patients will not knowingly risk their health or their life for the sake of "science." Every experienced clinical investigator knows this. When such risks are taken and a considerable number of patients are involved, it may be assumed that informed consent has not been obtained in all cases.

The gain anticipated from an experiment must be commensurate with the risk involved.

An experiment is ethical or not at its inception; it does not become ethical post hoc—ends do not justify means. There is no ethical distinction between ends and means. (86)

## General Impact of Controlled Clinical Trials on Medical Practice

While the clinical trial does not affect medical practice precisely in the way its proponents claim, in a different sense it does exert a profound and pernicious effect in determining the types of medicines which the pharmaceutical industry is inclined to develop.

In a word, the requirement that the drug pass the obstacle course of the controlled clinical trial favors nonspecific medicines over specific ones. And this inherent doctrinal or scientific impulse is reinforced by the economics of the drug market.

Because the medicine undergoing trial is not specifically adapted to any one individual but must exert its effect on a non-homogeneous group, it must seek to influence the metabolism over a broad spectrum of functions. In this it is bolstered by biological thinking generally, which has concentrated on general metabolic processes common to all species.

Rene Dubos has described this tendency very well:

Most of biological, physiological, and biochemical research has been focussed so far on the study of the phenomena which are common to all living things ... the largest achievement of modern biochemistry has been the demonstration of the fundamental *unity* of the chemical processes associated with life ... While this so-called fundamental approach has been immensely fruitful for the discovery of the structures and reactions which are *common* to all forms of life, it has almost completely failed to provide information concerning the structures and reactions which determine the *peculiarities* of each organ and function. As a result, the search for metabolic inhibitors has been limited to attempts at interfering with processes ubiquitous in all living things, for the simple reason that these are the only ones which are known. (Rene Dubos, Ph.D., 1964)(87)

The methodologic weaknesses of the clinical trial reinforce this tendency of biological thought, leading to a preference for non-specific medicines tested in large doses. The less specific the medicine, and the larger the dose, the more likely that everyone in the test sample will manifest some sort of response, papering over a degree of inhomogeneity. Hence clinical trials are biased in favor of large doses of nonspecific medicines.* (88)

Furthermore, the manufacturer has a strong economic inducement to favor drugs of broad application. He can recoup the enormous costs of the clinical trials needed for FDA approval—which can run as high as $50 million or more — only if his product is later marketed for a variety of different disease conditions. (89)

Hence, when the drug has been approved for sale, the manufacturer tries to include as many indications as possible on the package insert:

> To a guy in a drug house who is writing the promotional literature for the drug, *interpretation* may mean life or death for that drug in the marketplace.
>
> This can be one of the major causes of delay [in the FDA]. Everything is set, there is no disagreement that this is a safe and effective drug; now, how broad is the licence to advertise? The package insert is a critical question for the drug house. They must fight to get the broadest interpretation consistent with the data. The FDA people rightly feel that they must put this in proper perspective. The key to it is face-to-face discussion with interested parties and consultants. The meeting won't take an hour, but it shouldn't take two years. (David Rall, M.D., 1971)(90)

It can be plausibly maintained that the high incidence of adverse reactions to drugs in modern industrialized societies reflects the use of non-specific medicines instead of specific and, ultimately, the impact of the controlled clinical trial on the choice of pharmacologic substances for development.

---

*The meaning of "specificity" is discussed at length in the author's *Divided Legacy: a History of the Schism in Medical Thought* (H. Coulter, 1975, 1977).

## An Alternative: the Orphan Drug Paradigm

But is there an alternative? Can pharmacological substances be developed other than in reliance on the "general laws of biology"? Reference may be made again to the concept of "idiosyncrasy," meaning the essential wholeness or individuality of the individual. While "idiosyncrasy" is impossible to define using the known laws of biology or physiology (if it were so definable, it would no longer be "idiosyncrasy"), every physician has encountered it.

The idiosyncratic differences among patients, presumably of genetic origin, are what make patient samples heterogeneous and undermine the theory and practice of the clinical trial.

The biological or physiological determinants of idiosyncrasy are not known and remain to be discovered. They could be the object of biological and pharmacological research but are not. Therapeutic effort directed at the individual's idiosyncrasy is an unexplored alternative.

The pharmacologic counterpart of the patient's "idiosyncrasy" is the "specific medicine."

The meaning of "specificity" is also largely undefined, but Rene Dubos has given a good approximation:

> Powerful metabolic inhibitors have been synthesized on the basis of [general biological] knowledge, but in general they lack selectivity. Being directed against fundamental processes, they affect many different biological functions and are therefore likely to exhibit various forms of toxicity which sharply limit their usefulness. It is obvious that the sharper the selectivity of a biologically active substance, the greater the probability that it will be innocuous for cells and functions other than the one for which it has been designed. In other words, a substance is more likely to be therapeutically useful if it acts almost uniquely against a structure or an activity peculiar to the organism or function to be affected. *Unfortunately, the*

*physiological or chemical definition of these specific structures and activities is an aspect of biology which is grossly neglected at the present time....* [added] (Rene Dubos, Ph.D., 1964)(91)

Just as "non-specific" medicines are necessarily associated with a high incidence of adverse reactions, so the more "specific" medicine, with "sharper selectivity," will presumably have a lower incidence of adverse reactions. This line of research should be pursued.

This truth was obliquely recognized in the 1980s by professional and official adoption of the concept of the "orphan drug," also known as the "public service" or "limited-use" drug and meaning one employed in a disease affecting fewer than 200,000 individuals.

While the orphan drug is not precisely the same as the "highly specific" drug, there are many parallels between them, and the procedures developed for approving and licensing the former could well be applied to the latter.

It is difficult or impossible to assemble enough patients to perform clinical trials on orphan drugs, and, because the market is too small, the major drug companies are not interested in developing them:

Suppose you were in charge of research planning at a company and some scientist came along and said, "Gee, I have a great idea for a drug that would be useful for X disease" — which is not a very common disease. You ask, "What is the ultimate market?" He says, "A few thousand patients a year." You ask, "How much money do you think we might make on it per year?" and he gives you a very small figure. You ask, "What is your estimate of how much it would cost us and how long it would take to get the drug approved?" He says, "It would take us a fantastic amount of money and years of work." Then you say, "Let's forget that one." (Louis Lasagna, M.D., 1971)(92)

No company wants to spend $50 to $100 million obtaining FDA approval for a drug with limited application, and expedited procedures have sometimes been found. The representative of the CIBA Corporation told a drug-industry gathering in 1970 how one such drug — desferioxamine, for treating iron poisoning in children — got the go-ahead:

> This drug would probably still be in FDA if it weren't for [FDA Commissioner Herbert Ley]. We spent well over a million dollars to develop it. The gross sales run around $35,000 a year. One of the monitors at the FDA was reading the letter of the law very carefully. He said we had to do controlled studies, which is ridiculous. Finally, Dr. Cohn, our Medical Director, went to Herb and discussed the problem. It was quite obvious; Herb just signed the letter... It was essentially quite clear ... the whole situation was tied up because of lack of clear understanding or following the letter of the law so exactly that it didn't permit the individual to make an obvious decision. (George de Stevens, M.D., 1971)(93)

In 1983 the Congress passed the "Orphan Drug Act," which grants drug manufacturers a 73% tax writeoff of the cost of conducting clinical trials of such drugs and provides for a procedure which will be adapted to the specific features of each such drug, taking into consideration the small number of patients who may be available for testing. About 2000 drugs are thought to be affected.

A.B.Hill, the father of the controlled clinical trial, stated in the end of his life:

> Given the right attitude of mind there is more than one way in which we can study therapeutic efficacy. Any belief that the controlled trial is the only way would mean, not that the pendulum had swung too far, but that it had come right off the hook. (A.B. Hill, 1971)(94)

The evolving orphan drug procedure may be an alternative which is applicable also to drugs of higher specificity, thus enabling the pendulum to be put back on the hook.

## Socioeconomic Function of the Clinical Trial

The controlled clinical trial has little or no medical justification, but it has one clear socioeconomic function in 20th-century American industrialized society: that of restricting the flow of new knowledge into medicine and of new medicines into commerce.

In this way it helps perpetuate the monopoly or quasi-monopoly position of the medical-industrial complex. (95)

Any monopoly hates innovations which upset existing production and marketing programs. If it can control and limit the input of new ideas (and in medicine new drugs are new ideas), it thereby reinforces its economic dominance. (96)

If innovation cannot be controlled, it becomes a loose cannon, crushing friend and foe alike.

This is especially dangerous in the drug industry which is marked by a high degree of product instability. When twenty industries were measured for "instability" in 1975, pharmaceutical manufacturing was found to be in the No. 2 position. And within a given therapeutic class, where drugs are interchangeable, a leading product can lose its dominance very rapidly after the appearance of a new one considered by the medical community to be safer and/or more effective. (97)

Drug-industry officials lie awake nights worrying about the new "Miracle-cillin" that may cut into sales of their own "cillin." Hence innovation must be kept within bounds. If the pipeline can be constricted so that outsiders are barred from the market and competition is limited to a small group of companies, officials will sleep that much better.

Innovation may be the lifeblood of the "brand-name" manufacturers, but it is heavily circumscribed. No one wants to see the market disarrayed by some maverick inventor curing cancer in his basement. The "efficacy" requirement helps prevent this from happening.

In the not-too-distant past medical innovation was due precisely to such lonely scientists working with patients and coming forward with new suggestions for treatment, but this avenue has now been closed off almost completely. While articles are still published detailing the experience and ideas of an individual practitioner, they are not regarded as sources of new discoveries. They do not appear in reputable journals and are not taken seriously by anyone. The practitioner has been relegated to the sidelines. The OTA *Background Report* comments:

> Traditionally, the physician has been the arbiter and judge of medical practices. It was presumed that careful observation about patients and reasoning about cause and effect would make the physician the best instrument to judge the success or failure of clinical practices. Until nearly the middle of this century, that presumption was largely unquestioned. (98)

The agents of innovation and change today are the drug manufacturers. They are the ones who decide which medicines are to be made available to the public.

The high cost of bringing a new medicine into the world — estimated at $200 million to $1 billion for a new molecular entity, and with 25% of that total allocated to clinical trials, toxicity studies, bioavailability studies and the other exercises needed for FDA approval — means that only companies which can afford the price of admission can join the game.*(99)

The clinical trial, with its accompanying financial pressure, favors large corporations over small — established businesses over would-be new entries. And since the FDA's requirements are stricter than those of any other country, foreigners wishing to sell in the U.S. market must comply with these more rigid standards. The monopoly position of U.S. drug manufacturers is thereby extended beyond this country's borders. (100)

---

*In 1979 the Eli Lilly Co. only needed data on 1493 patients to obtain FDA approval for its oral antimicrobial *Ceclor*. By 1989 a new antimicrobial required data on 10,000 patients. A New Drug Application in the 1940s could be carried in a briefcase; in 1988 the NDA for Eli Lilly's *Permax* weighed two tons and contained 320 million words. (Institute for Alternative Futures: Seminar, December 11, 1989)

The necessity of conducting trials also affords drug manufacturers a way to purchase the services and loyalties of physicians and professors of medicine. Advancement in the medical school hierarchy is a function of publications, and the clinical trial is a source of publications:

> The clinical trial has become the latest in a long line of medical status symbols. It has become a political instrument and a mechanism for career development. (Bernard Fisher, M.D., 1983)(101)

The clinical trial ideal is wielded as a weapon especially against unconventional (alternative) modes of therapy — lonely physician-inventors working in their garages — who may not be willing to sell their ideas to one of the large manufacturers. These physicians are told blandly by the FDA that their therapies do not measure up to "scientific" standards, even though these standards are not attained by anyone else. At the same time, drugs from more favored suppliers can be exempted from the testing requirements by a mere letter from the FDA Commissioner.

Since the treatment of cancer in the United States today is a $1 billion industry, unorthodox or "unrecognized" cancer therapies are in particular disfavor. These physicians are admonished for failure to perform trials following the paradigm outlined in the above pages, then branded as "quacks" and turned over to the police. But the discerning critics in the FDA and the American Cancer Society apply a more stringent rule to "unorthodox" physicians than they do to their own grant recipients. Cancer is known to be a highly heterogeneous disease, with any sample composed of numerous subsets differing significantly from one another. Conventional drug trials in cancer are nearly always conducted with very small patient samples, and, in fact, are criticized for this. But unorthodox practitioners are cited as "unscientific" for doing the same. The ire directed at "unorthodox" cancer therapies has little to do with the supposed scientific inadequacies of these therapies. Rather the contrary: the more promising the idea, the more likely it is to end up on the

American Cancer Society's list, "Unproven Methods of Cancer Management."* A genuine advance would seriously disrupt this billion-dollar market. (102)

The ordinary observer might assume that the treatments on this list have been demonstrated ineffective. That is not the case: they have not been subjected to any testing at all — neither by the American Cancer Society nor by any other agency, public or private. They merely *seem* ineffective in the light of prevailing theories of cancer etiology and therapy. But no procedure on this list will ever obtain the financing or bureaucratic approval needed to demonstrate its therapeutic value. Hence, characterizing a cancer therapy as "unproven" is a self-fulfilling prophecy in the truest sense of the word. Competition by maverick researchers is effectively suppressed.

A large proportion of the personnel and facilities available for clinical trials is used to test so-called "me too" drugs — the copy-cat molecules which emerge when Company A sees that Company B's new diuretic is doing well in the marketplace and decides to produce a knock-off. (103) Companies often prefer to steal market share from competitors — rather than create a new product to meet an imperfectly defined demand. (104)

> Given the scarcity of resources (funds, staff, and patients) for conducting randomized clinical trials we must be concerned about many "me too" drugs that occupy these resources solely for proprietary reasons. (Michael Bracken, M.D., 1987)(105)

---

*The Coley Vaccines were on this list for decades, and then discovered to be effective after all (R.G.Houston, 11). Immunological treatments were branded "quackery" in the 1950s and then recognized as promising in the 1980s. How many patients have been deprived of their lives in the meantime — because officials of the American Cancer Society (who may have graduated from medical school forty years earlier) do not understand a new approach to cancer therapy?

The "me too" drug is purely and simply an instrument for increasing drug-company profitability and may be of little or no marginal benefit to society. How many diuretics, after all, does a country need?

The socio-economic impact of the Kefauver-Harris Amendments has been precisely the opposite of what Estes Kefauver wanted.

It will be recalled that his famous Hearings were entitled: *Study of Administered Prices in the Drug Industry*. His purpose was economic: to compel the drug industry to lower drug prices by promoting competition between "brand-name" and "generic" drugs. Since the major pharmaceutical manufacturers had always charged that "generic" drugs were of inferior quality, Kefauver's initial draft legislation called on the FDA to ensure the "purity, safety, and efficacy" of all drugs. (106) In this way the U.S. consumer would have a choice between a "brand-name" and a "generic" drug of identical "purity, safety, and efficacy."*

Kefauver's intent, however, has been perverted. The FDA's hyper-rigid interpretation of the "efficacy" provision, rather than ensuring comparability of "brand-name" and "generic" drugs and thus lowering the price to the consumer, grants an effective monopoly to the large drug companies. New drug entities, which are traditionally the most profitable, are very largely the province of these manufacturers.

Hence the latter form a powerful constituency for the controlled clinical trial — which is a reliable guarantor of their continuing profitability.

---

*This issue is still very much alive. In 1987 the *Journal of the American Medical Association* received and published an article purporting to find the "brand-name" anti-epileptic drug, *Mysoline*, superior to its generic version, primidone. The trial was in a single patient, and publication of the article had a "decidedly negative impact" on sales of primidone. Later it was discovered that the patient's status deteriorated on *Mysoline* as well, and she had to be switched to other anti-epileptics. This information was known a year before the article was published but was never communicated to the AMA. (D. Rennie, 1989)

In 1969 the association of generic manufacturers warned of increasing oligopoly in the drug industry due to the soaring costs of demonstrating drug efficacy. (107) This did indeed come to pass, and the Pharmaceutical Manufacturers' Association (representing "brand-name" manufacturers) noted with satisfaction in 1980:

> By any number of measures of research and invention, including the size of R & D budgets and the innovational output of the largest firms, there has been a trend towards fewer companies successfully engaging in new product development. (108)

The number of drug companies in the United States fell from 1114 in 1958 to 756 in 1972. (109) During the years 1959-1962 an average of 109 firms per year were introducing new pharmaceutical products. For the years 1971 through 1977 the average had dropped to 47. (110)

Monopolies are congenitally hostile to the innovation which is the major dynamic of economic progress. Hence monopolistic or semi-monopolistic control of the marketplace has traditionally been censured in the United States — witness passage of the Sherman and Clayton antitrust acts in the late nineteenth century and the ongoing activity of the Antitrust Division of the Department of Justice.

If the controlled clinical trial were recognized for what it is — a mainstay of drug-industry and medical-industrial-complex monopoly — the antitrust impulse in American society would be directed against it today.

The interests of the Pharmaceutical Manufacturers' Association may often be in conflict with the good health of Americans. The controlled clinical trial benefits primarily the balance-sheets of the major drug manufacturers. Who is to say that the medicines best adapted to improving drug-company balance sheets are always likely to ameliorate the public's health?

This tragic situation need never have happened. The Kefauver-Harris Amendments speak only of "adequate and well-controlled investigations, including clinical investigations." The FDA, which gave these amendments its own particular spin, could reverse course at will and thus eliminate many of the negative features discussed in the above pages.

## Conclusion

The OTA *Background Paper* on clinical trials notes that: "objections are rarely if ever raised to the principles of controlled experimentation on which RCTs are based." (111) Our analysis has aimed to do precisely that. We consider the controlled clinical trial to be a wrongheaded attempt by man to subjugate nature. Its advocates hope to overcome the innate and ineluctable heterogeneity of the human species in both sickness and health merely by applying a rigid procedure.

In Chapter I we observed: "the intractable problem which the clinical trial is supposed to resolve is that of human variety." But the obstacle of human variety is not actually overcome by the clinical trial. It is merely assumed out of existence.

While this effort may represent a sort of utopian impulse, a yen for perfectability, utopias have a way of turning into their opposites. And this has happened with the controlled clinical trial. Far from improving medical practice, it has had the opposite effect: (1) it helps perpetuate the monopoly or semi-monopoly of the major pharmaceutical manufacturers at the expense of small drug companies and individual practitioners; (2) it helps raise the price of drugs and medical services; and (3) it contributes to the present high incidence of acute illness, chronic disease, and death from "side effects" of the powerful and non-specific drugs necessarily spawned by such a system.

The trial rests on the unverified assumption that the "normal biological diversity" of human beings is a negligible factor in medicine. The preceding pages have demonstrated this factor to be far from negligible. Indeed, it has survived all attempts to subjugate it and remains the Achilles' heel of the clinical trial procedure.

The entire $550 billion American medical industry revolves to some degree around the controlled clinical trial. But, because the theory is defective, the enormous superstructure erected upon it is equally shaky. The effect has been simply to raise costs all around and thus to limit the efficacy of society's expenditures in this area.

The American public should at length come to realize that medicine ("health care," as it is called) consumes over 11% of the U.S. gross national product every year, and that purely scientific considerations will always yield in the confrontation with this sort of economic might. Belief that late 20th-century medicine is oriented mainly toward scientific goals is mere self-delusion.

While the clinical trial may have a role to play, it is ludicrous to fit all pharmacological development to the dimensions of this procrustean bed. Aside from the theoretical and practical defects noted in the above pages, it is a very expensive way of discovering information — probably too expensive, in the long run, even for the United States:

> Clinical trials pose a challenge to NIH because the number of significant questions that can be answered through clinical trials clearly exceeds our ability — indeed, the nation's — to plan, execute, and finance all the studies that are needed. (Donald S. Fredrickson, M.D., 1979)(112)

Surgical and other "procedures" used in modern medical practice are rarely (only 10% to 20% of the time) verified by controlled clinical trials. (113) And yet, therapeutic catastrophes do not occur more commonly there.

At the same time, the incidence of adverse reactions, iatrogenic diseases, and subsequent chronic disease from the use and abuse of the non-specific drugs generated by the clinical trial process shows no sign of abating.

Chronic disease is this country's major health problem. (114)

If the medicines used in today's practice are to be better adapted to the specific features of patients, their idiosyncrasies, and thus less likely to generate the myriad "side effects" with which we are only too lamentably familiar, they will have to be developed following principles other than those of the controlled clinical trial.

# NOTES

## INTRODUCTION

1. Silverman, M. *et al.*, 34.
2. Stone, G.B., 336.
3. *Ibid.*, 327.
4. Silverman, M. *et al.*, 38, 327.PMA, 1980a, 7; 1990, 5.
5. *Ibid.*, 38, 124.
6. Vandenbroucke, Jan P., 985.
7. Atkins, H., 377.
8. U.S.Congress. Office of Technology Assessment, 1983, 32.
9. *Ibid.*, 33.
10. *W.Post*, March 8, 1978, A-1.
11. *New York Times*, December 8, 1987, C-3.
12. Blum, A.L. *et al.*
13. Bracken, Michael B., 1111.

## I.  HUMAN VARIETY IN HEALTH AND DISEASE

1. Quoted in Coulter, H.L., 1975, 262.
2. Williams, R., 1957-1958, 98-99.
3. *Ibid.*, 100.
4. Cooper, J. D., 1971b, 94.
5. Linder, Maria C., 114-115.

6. American Society of Hospital Pharmacists, 100. Sodeman, W.A. and W.A.,Jr., 202-203.

7. Kabat, Elvin, A., 8.

8. Fudenburg, H.H. *et al.*, 3.

9. Dubos, Rene, 1970, 183.

10. *New York Times*, November 2, 1971.

11. Nodine, J.H. and Siegler, P.E., 16.

12. *New York Times*, November 2, 1971.

13. *Loc. cit.*

14. *Loc. cit.*

15. Goodman, A.G., *et al.*, 1148.

16. Linder, Maria C., 143.

17. Nodine, J.H. *et al.*, 13, 18-19.

18. Williams, R., 1957-1958, 100.

19. National Analysts, 84.

20. Talalay, Paul, ed., 93-94.

## II.  THE DISEASE ENTITY

1. USDHEW PHS, 1976.

2. Faber, Knud, 63.

3. Herrick, A.D. *et al.*, 132.

4. Witts, L.J., 7, 13.

5. Quoted in Faber, Knud, 27.

6. Witts, L.J., 7.

7. Herrick, A.D. *et al.*, 132.

8. Feinstein, A., 1976, 101-102.

9. Feinstein, A., 1977, 363.

10. Feinstein, A., 1976, 69, 212.

11. *Ibid.*, 69.

12. Witts, L.J., 37.

13. Feinstein, A., 1976, 69.

14. *Loc. cit.*

15. Osler, W., 841.

16. Ross, O.B., Jr., 35. See, also, American Society of Hospital Pharmacists, 94; Harvey, A. McGhehee *et al.*, 203, 344.

17. Feinstein, A., 1976, 68. Herfindal, E.T. *et al.*, 155, 157. American Society of Hospital Pharmacists, 97. Ross, O.B., Jr., 35.

18. Witts, L.J., 37.

19. Feinstein, A., 1976, 91.

20. *Ibid.*, 68, 92.

21. *Ibid.*, 68.

22. *Ibid.*, 83-84, 126. See, also, Witts, L.J., 26.

23. Vickers, G., 1024.

24. Feinstein, A., 1976, 100-101.

25. Emanuel, Elliott, 1234.

26. *New York Times*, June 17, 1982.

27. Kapit, R.M., 207. Wing, J. *et al.*

28. Herrick, A.D. *et al.*, 132.

29. Hoffer, Abram, 1960-1961, 221-222.

30. *New York Times*, November 13, 1979, C-2.

31. Hollister, L.E. *et al.*, 486.

32. Hoffer, Abram, 1960-1961, 221-222.

33. *Washington Post*, May 20, 1982.

34. Ropes, Marian W., 1956.

35. Committee Report, 1963. Harvey, A. McGhehee *et al.*, 1406.

36. American Psychiatric Association, 1987, 224.

37. Vickers, G., 1026.

38. Sodeman, W.A. and W.A., Jr., 3.

39. Thomas, Lewis, 1972, 52.

40. Feinstein, A., 1976, 333.

41. *Ibid.*, 92.

42. *Ibid.*, 331.

43. Perkins, W.H., 21-23.

44. Feinstein, A., 1979, 488.

45. Feinstein, A., 1976, 84.

46. *Ibid.*, 100.

## III. HOMOGENEITY vs. GENERALIZABILITY

1. Herrick, A.D. *et al.*, 129.

2. Feinstein, A., 1977, 155.

3. Herrick, A.D. *et al.*, 129.

4. Beveridge, W.I.B., 20, 28.

5. Platt, R., 1963, 1158.

6. *Lancet*, 1964 (ii), October 31, 949.

7. Hill, A.B., 1966, 108.

8. Brown, B.W., Jr., 19.

9. Thomson, M.E. *et al.*, 295.

10. Evans, M. *et al.*, 110.

11. Gifford, R.H. *et al.*, 351.

12. Institute on Drug Literature Evaluation, 74.

13. Hoffer, Abram, 1967, 124.

14. Johnson, F.N. *et al.*, 132.

15. Modell, Walter, 1960, 770.

16. Hill, A.B., ed., 1960, 21.

17. Witts, L.J., 32.

18. Johnson, F.N. *et al.*, 47-48.

19. Yerushalmy, J. *et al.*, 1950. Yerushalmy, J. *et al.*, 1 9 5 1 . Fletcher, C.M.

20. Witts, L.J., 42-49.

21. Mondzac, A.M.

22. Whittlesey, M., 126.

23. Feinstein, A., 1976, 91.

24. Siegler, E.E. See, also, Belk, W.P. *et al.*

25. Gordis, Leon.

26. DeGowin, E.L. *et al.*, 7.

27. Bakwin, Harry.

28. U.S. Congress, Office of Technology Assessment, 1983,79.

29. Spence, James, 630.

30. "Dr. Weed Sounds Off for POMR," *Medical Group News* (July, 1974), 3-5.

31. Johnson, F.N. *et al.*, 177.

32. Cooper, J.D., ed., 1971b, 59, 62.

33. Johnson, F.N. *et al.*, 39-40.

34. Meyer, J.L.

35. Northrop, F.S.C., 1960: Chapter III.

36. Herrick, A.D. *et al.*, 129.

37. McPeek, B., 724.

38. Feinstein, A., 1977, 171.

39. Herrick, A.D. *et al.*, 134.

40. Feinstein, A., 1977, 23.

41. Feinstein, A., 1976, 214-225; Herrick, A.D. *et al.*, 130-135; Harris, E.L. *et al.*, 54.

42. Weiss, W. *et al.*, 678.

43. Brown, George W.; Roberts, Robin, *et al.*; Feinstein, A., 1979.

44. Herrick, A.D. *et al.*, 134. Canner, P. L., 1979, 659.

45. Dupont, W.D., 940.

46. Lawrence K. Altman, "AIDS Virus: Always Fatal?" *New York Times*, September 8, 1987. John Lauritsen, "Kangaroo Court Etiology," *New York Native*, May 8, 1988, 8. Darrow, W.H. *et al.* Coulter, H. 1987, 1990.

## IV. SAMPLE SIZE, RANDOMIZATION, STRATIFICATION

1. Gordon, R.S., Jr. Clark, C.J. *et al.* Fredrickson, D.S., 1968, 992-993.

2. Chassan, J.B., 174.

3. Cooper, J.B., 1971b, 156.

4. Brown, B.W., Jr., 22-23.

5. Feinstein, A., 1977, 11.

6. Cooper, J.D., 1971b, 271.

7. Feinstein, A., 1977, 10-11.

8. Johnson, F.N. *et al.*, 54.

9. Grizzle, J.E., 365.

10. *Loc. cit.* Johnson, F.N. *et al.*, 65.

11. U.S.Congress, Office of Technology Assessment, 1983, 9.

12. Herrick, A.D. *et al.*, 135.

13. Angell, Marcia, 1385. See, also, Taylor, K.M. *et al.* and Spodick, D.H.

14. Chalmers, T. C., 291.

15. Mackillop, W.J. *et al.*, 185.

16. Angell, Marcia, 1386-1387.

17. Meier, P., 361.

18. Fisher, B., 69-70.

19. Johnson, F.N. *et al.*, 79.

20. U.S.Congress. Office of Technology Assessment, 1983, 54.

21. Johnson, F.N. *et al.*, 78. Harris, E.L. *et al.*, 43. Binns, T.B. *et al.*, 1150.

22. U.S.Congress, Office of Technology Assessment, 1983, 54.

23. Collins, J.F. *et al.*, 228.

24. *Loc. cit.*

25. U.S.Congress. Office of Technology Assessment, 1983, 54.

26. Hoffer, A., 1967, 124.

27. Green, S.B., 190-191.

28. *Loc. cit.*

29. Dupont, W.D., 942.

30. Meinert, C.L., 249.

31. U.S.Congress. Office of Technology Assessment, 1983, 54. Tannock, Ian *et al.*, 67.

32. Witts, L.J., 33. Harris, E.L. *et al.*, 56.

33. Johnson, F.N. *et al.*, 44.

34. *Loc. cit.*

35. Feinstein, A., 1976, 224-225.

36. U.S.Congress. Office of Technology Assessment, 1983, 53. Institute for Alternative Futures: Seminar, December 11, 1989.

37. Harris, E.L. *et al.*, 43-46.

## V.   MEASUREMENT. DEFINING CURE

1. Johnson, F.N. *et al.*, 39.

2. Cooper, J.D., ed., 1971b, 72.

3. Johnson, F.N. *et al.*, 46.

4. Feinstein, A., 1976, 139.

5. Johnson, F.N. *et al.*, 48.

6. Feinstein, A., 1976, 61. See, also, Cromie, B.W., 994; Hill, A.B., 1960, 20.

7. Cooper, J.D., ed., 1971b, 70. See, also, Feinstein, A., 1976, 84; Hill, A.B., ed., 1960, 26.

8. Hutchinson, T.A. *et al.*

9. Johnson, F.N.*et al.*, 48.

10. Cromie, B.W., 996.

11. Ritchie, D.M. *et al.*, 405. Harris, E.L. *et al.*, 126.

12. Feinstein, A., 1976, 36.

13. Feinstein, A., 1977, 10. Brown, B. W., Jr., 23.

14. Feinstein, A., 1976, 255.

15. Hill, A.B., 1960, 26.

16. Rutstein, D. 108.

17. *Physicians' Desk Reference*, 1989, 2282.

18. Cooper, J.D., ed., 1971b, 9.

19. Ross, O.B., Jr., 35-36.

20. Beeson, Paul B. *et al.*, 1001.

21. *Physicians' Desk Reference*, 1989, 2178.

22. Cooper, J.D., ed., 1971b, 65.

23. Feinstein, A., 1976, 41, 44.

24. *Ibid.*, 65.

25. *Loc. cit.*

26. Hoffer, A., 1967, 124. Dupont, W.D., 942.

27. Palmer, R., ed., 14.

28. American Society of Hospital Pharmacists, 177-178.

29. Harris, E.L. *et al.*,115.

30. Cooper, J.D., 1971b, 51.

31. *Ibid.*, 33.

32. Bracken, M.B., 1111.

33. Jones, Hardin B., 331.

34. Abel, U. See, also, *Der Spiegel,* 33/1990, 174-176.

35. Feinstein, A., 1977, 10-11.

# VI. THE DOUBLE BLIND. CONDUCT OF THE CLINICAL TRIAL

1. Hoffer, Abram, 1967, 123.

2. Johnson, F.N. *et al.*, 67, 73.

3. Hoffer, Abram, 1967, 125.

4. Johnson, F.N. *et al.*, 74. Fligor, L.W.

5. Moscucci, M. *et al.*, 264.

6. Johnson, F.N. *et al.*, 74.

7. U.S.Congress. Office of Technology Assessment, 1983, 52.

8. Johnson, F.N. *et al.*, 74.

9. *Loc. cit.*

10. *Loc. cit.* Hoffer, Abram, 1967, 125.

11. Moscucci, M. *et al.*, 259.

12. Levine, R.J., 247, 249.

13. Harris, E.L. *et al.*, 56.

14. Banta, H.D., 175.

15. Johnson, F.N. *et al.*, 49, 50.

16. Brown, B.W., Jr., 17. Meier, Paul, 360.

17. DeMets, D.L. *et al.*

18. Wade, N.

19. Cooper, J.D., ed., 1971a, 83. Vonderhaar, T.A. *et al.*, 54.

20. Gifford, R.H. *et al. New York Times*, August 28, 1980.

21. *Washington Post*, June 8, 1969, A-9. U.S.Senate. Select Committee on Small Business. Subcommittee on Monopoly, Part 11, February-March, 1969, 4496.

22. Cooper, J.D., ed., 1971a, 89.
23. Palmer, R., ed., 14.
24. Vonder Haar, T.A. *et al.*, 54.
25. *Loc. cit.*
26. *Loc. cit.*
27. Special Committee on Internal Pollution, 509.
28. Shapiro, M.F. *et al.*, 2505-2506.
29. Lisook, A.B.
30. U.S.Senate. Select Committee on Small Business. Subcommittee on Monopoly, Part 11, February-March, 1969, 4493.
31. Lisook, A.B.
32. *New York Times*, July 21, 1976, 8.
33. *Washington Post*, March 8, 1978, A-10.
34. *Washington Star*, March 8, 1978.
35. *Washington Post*, October 12, 1979, A-3.
36. *New York Times*, October 30, 1987, 1, D-24. *Wall Street Journal*, May 19, 1989, B-4.
37. NOVA
38. Cruzan, S.
39. NOVA
40. Wade, N.
41. Shapiro, M.F. *et al.*, 2509.
42. *Ibid.*, 2508.
43. *Ibid.*,2507, 2509.
44. *Ibid.*, 2508

45. U.S.Senate. Select Committee on Small Business, Subcommittee on Monopoly, Part II, February-March, 1969, 4491, 4493.

46. Wade, N.

47. Pfeifer, Mark P. *et al.*

# VII. STATISTICAL ANALYSIS

1. Feinstein, A., 1977, 9, 11.

2. Harris, E.L. *et al.*, 113, 116.

3. Tannock, Ian *et al.*, 67. See, also, J.D.Cooper, ed., 1971b, 16.

4. NOVA

5. Feinstein, A., 1977, 11.

6. Maxwell, C.

7. U.S.Congress. Office of Technology Assessment, 1983, 46.

8. Harris, E.L. *et al.*, 125.

9. Cooper, J.D., ed., 1971b, 168.

# VIII. THE CLINICAL TRIAL: FOR OR AGAINST?

1. Northrop, F.S.C., 35.

2. *Ibid.*, 38.

3. Cooper, J.D., ed., 1971b, 64.

4. Hill, A.B., 1966, 109.

5. "Dr. Weed Sounds Off for POMR." *Medical Group News*, July, 1974, 3.

6. Feinstein, A., 1976, 71, 126.
7. Friedman, H.S.
8. Mackillop, W.J. *et al.*, 186.
9. Binns, T.B., *et al.*, 1150.
10. Cooper, J.D., ed., 1971b, 16.
11. Grizzle, J.E., 365.
12. Fredrickson, D.S., 1979, 631.
13. Platt, R., 1158.
14. Friedman, H.S.
15. Browne, B.W.,Jr., 22.
16. Dupont, W.D., 940. Fredrickson, D.S., 1979, 630.
17. Fredrickson, D.S., 1968, 986. See, also, Horwitz, R.I., 96, and Friedman, H.S.
18. Cooper, J.D., ed., 1971b, 272-273.
19. Horwitz, R.I., 93.
20. *Loc. cit.*
21. Miller, S.T. *et al.*, 534.
22. Bracken, M.B., 1112.
23. Cooper, J.D., ed., 1971a, 181.
24. *New York Times*, August 28, 1980.
25. Friedman, H.S.
26. *Loc. cit.*
27. *New York Times*, April 15, 1990, E-5.
28. *Washington Post*, January 21, 1976.
29. Vonderhaar, T.A. *et al.*, 46.
30. *Ibid.*, 48.

31. *Physicians' Desk Reference*, 1989, 1988.

32. *Ibid.*, 1989.

33. Canner, P.L., 1983, 274.

34. Quoted in U.S.Congress. Office of Technology Assessment, 1983, 75.

35. *Physicians' Desk Reference*, 1989, 2282.

36. Friedman, L. *et al.*, 519.

37. *Physicians' Desk Reference*, 1989, 2282.

38. *New York Times*, September 20, 1973, 20.

39. *Loc. cit.*

40. *Washington Post*, August 22, 1985.

41. U.S.Congress. Office of Technology Assessment, 1983, 50.

42. *Loc. cit.*

43. *Washington Post*, May 28, 1990, A-4.

44. U.S.Senate. Committee on Labor and Public Welfare. Subcommittee on Health, Part 5, May 20, 1974, 1545.

45. Steel, Knight *et al.*, 638.

46. H.D.R., Jr. D'Arcy, P.F. *et al.*

47. USDHHS PHS, 1988, 93. Strauss, A., *passim.*

48. The WHO study is cited in Lasagna, L., 1980, 5.

49. Cooper, J.D., ed., 1971b, 65.

50. Fredrickson, D.S., 1979, 630.

51. American Society of Hospital Pharmacists, 5-6.

52. Feinstein, A., 1976, 41.

53. U.S.Congress. Office of Technology Assessment, 1983, 62.

54. *Loc. cit.*

55. *Ibid.*, 61.

56. Bracken, M.B. 1112.

57. Blum, A.L. *et al.*

58. Fredrickson, D.S., 1979, 631. See, also, U.S. Congress. Office of Technology Assessment, 1983, 62.

59. *Physicians' Desk Reference*, 1989, 565.

60. Palmer, R., ed., 31.

61. Friedman, L. *et al.*, 514.

62. *Ibid.*, 516.

63. *Ibid.*, 519.

64. Tyson, J.E., 1984, 301.

65. Chalmers, T.C., 294-295.

66. Herbst, Arthur I., *et al.*

67. *Washington Post*, January 13, 1977; January 25, 1980, A-8.

68. *Washington Post*, March 11, 1990, A-4.

69. Chalmers, T.C., 295.

70. *Loc. cit.*

71. *New York Times*, October 22, 1970.

72. *Washington Post*, January 28, 1975.

73. Chalmers, T.C., 296.

74. Canadian Schizophrenia Foundation. A. Hoffer, 1967.

75. U.S.Congress. Office of Technology Assessment, 1983, 33.

76. Cooper, J.D., ed., 1971b, 54.

77. *New York Times*, July 20, 1975, 15.

78. Hill, A.B., 1966, 110.

79. Fletcher, R.H. and S.W., 182.

80. Hill, A.B., 1966, 110.

81. Palmer, R., 56.

82. Cooper, J.D., ed., 1971a, 65-66.

83. Palmer, R., ed,. 2-3.

84. *Ibid.*, 57.

85. *Daily Telegraph* (London), September 21, 1973.

86. Beecher, Henry K., 1360.

87. Talalay, Paul, ed., 39.

88. Harris, E.L. *et al.*, 61.

89. Hoffer, A., 1967, 125. Institute for Alternative Futures: Seminar, December 11, 1989.

90. Cooper, J.D., ed., 1971a, 95.

91. Talalay, Paul, ed., 39.

92. Cooper, J.D., ed., 1971a, 152.

93. *Ibid.*, 97-98.

94. Cooper, J.D., ed., 1971b, 11.

95. On the medical-industrial complex see A. Relman.

96. Moss, Ralph, Chapters 17 and 18.

97. Pharmaceutical Manufacturers' Association, 1980b, 52.

98. U.S.Congress. Office of Technology Assessment, 1983, 10.

99. Institute for Alternative Futures: Seminar, December 11, 1989.

100. Johnson, F.N. *et al.*, 200.

101. Fisher, B., 69.

102. *Loc. cit.* Tannock, I. *et al.* U.S.Congress. Office of Technology Assessment, 1983, 54. Houston, R.G. *passim.*

103. Bracken, M.B., 1111.

104. Institute for Alternative Futures: Seminar, December 11, 1989.

105. Bracken, M.B., 1111.

106. U.S.Senate. Select Committee on Small Business, Subcommittee on Monopoly, Part 11, February-March, 1969, 4478.

107. *Drug Trade News*, February 10, 1969.

108. Pharmaceutical Manufacturers' Association, 1980b, 50.

109. *Loc. cit.*

110. *Loc. cit.*

111. U.S.Congress. Office of Technology Assessment, 1983, 41.

112. Fredrickson, D.S., 1979, 630.

113. U.S.Congress. Office of Technology Assessment, 1978, 7.

114. Strauss, Anselm, 1.

# BIBLIOGRAPHY

Abel, Ulrich. *Chemotherapy of Advanced Epithelial Cancer.* Stuttgart: Hippokrates Verlag GmbH, 1990.

American Psychiatric Association, *Diagnostic and Statistical Manual.* Third Edition, Revised. Washington, D.C.: American Psychiatric Association, 1987.

American Society of Hospital Pharmacists, *Proceedings of the Institute on Drug Literature Evaluation.* Washington, D.C.: American Society of Hospital Pharmacists, 1969.

Angell, Marcia. "Patients' Preferences in Randomized Clinical Trials." *New England J.Med.* 310:21 (May 24, 1984), 1385-1387.

Armitage, Peter. "Importance of Prognostic Factors in the Analysis of Data from Clinical Trials." *Controlled Clinical Trials* I (1981), 347-353.

Atkins, Hedley. "Conduct of a Controlled Clinical Trial." *British M.J.* (August 13, 1966), 377-379.

Bakwin, Harry. "Pseudodoxia Pediatrica." *New England J. Med.* 232 (1945), 691-697.

Banta, H. David. "RCTs and the Federal Government." *Controlled Clinical Trials* 3 (1982), 173-183.

Beecher, Henry K. "Ethics and Clinical Research." *New England J. Med.* 274:24 (June 16, 1966), 1354-1360.

Beeson, Paul B. and Walsh McDermott. *Textbook of Medicine.* Two Volumes. Fourteenth Edition. Philadelphia: W.B.Saunders, 1975.

Belk, W.P. and F.W.Sunderman. "A Survey of the Accuracy of Chemical Analyses in Clinical Laboratories." *A.J.Clinical Pathology* 17 (1947), 853-861.

Beveridge, W.I.B. *The Art of Scientific Investigation*. New York: Vintage, 1957.

Binns, T.B. and Butterfield, W.J.H. "Clinical Trials: Some Constructive Suggestions." *Lancet* (May 23, 1964), 1150-1152.

Blum, A.L. *et al*. "The Lugano Statements on Controlled Clinical Trials." *The Journal of International Medical Research* 15 (1987), 2-22.

Bracken, Michael B. "Clinical Trials and the Acceptance of Uncertainty." *British Med. J.* (May 2, 1987), 1111-1112.

Brown, Byron W., Jr. "Statistical Controversies in the Design of Clinical Trials — Some Personal Views." *Controlled Clinical Trials* I (1980), 13-27.

Brown, George W. "Berkson Fallacy Revisited: Spurious Conclusions from Patient Surveys." *A. J. Dis. Child.* 130 (January, 1976), 5660.

Canadian Schizophrenia Foundation. *Megavitamin Therapy*. Regina: Canadian Schizophrenia Foundation, 1976.

Canner, Paul L. "Brief Description of the Coronary Drug Project and Other Studies." *Controlled Clinical Trials* 4 (1983), 273-280.

_____."Responses." *Clinical Pharm. and Ther.* 25:5 (Part 2) (May, 1979), 657-660.

Chalmers, Thomas C. "A Potpourri of RCT Topics." *Controlled Clinical Trials* 3 (1982), 285-298.

Chassan, J.B. "Statistical Inference and the Single Case in Clinical Design." *Psychiatry* 23 (1960), 173-184.

Clark, C.J. *et al.* "A Method for the Rapid Determination of the Number of Patients to Include in a Controlled Clinical Trial." *Lancet* 1966 (ii), 1357-1358.

Collins, Joseph F. *et al.* "Some Adaptive Strategies for Inadequate Sample Acquisition in Veterans Administration Cooperative Clinical Trials." *Controlled Clinical Trials* I (1980), 227-248.

"Committee Report — Jones Criteria (Revised) for Guidance in the Diagnosis of Rheumatic Fever." *Circulation* 32 (October, 1963), 664-668.

Cooper, Joseph D., ed. *Philosophy and Technology of Drug Assessment. Volume I. Decision-Making on the Efficacy and Safety of Drugs.* Washington, D.C.: Interdisciplinary Communication Associates, 1971a.

_____.Volume III. *The Philosophy of Evidence.* Washington, D. C.: Interdisciplinary Communication Associates, 1971b.

Coulter, Harris L. *Divided Legacy: A History of the Schism in Medical Thought. Volume I. The Patterns Emerge, Hippocrates to Paracelsus.* Washington, D.C.: Wehawken Book Company, 1975. *Volume II. Progress and Regress: J.B. Van Helmont to Claude Bernard.* Washington,D.C.: Wehawken Book Co., 1977.

_____. *AIDS and Syphilis: the Hidden Link.* Berkeley: North Atlantic Books, 1987. Second Edition. New Delhi: Jain, 1990.

Cromie, B.W. "The Feet of Clay of the Double-Blind Trial." *Lancet* 1963 (ii), 994-997.

Cruzan, Susan. "New Jersey Doctor Pleads Guilty to Drug Testing Fraud." FDA Talk Paper, October 25, 1988.

D'Arcy, P.F. and Griffin, J.P. *Iatrogenic Diseases*. London: Oxford University Press, 1972.

Darrow, W.H. *et al.* "Risk Factors for Human Immunodeficiency Virus (HIV) Infections in Homosexual Men." *A.J.Public Health* 77:4 (April, 1987), 479-483.

DeGowin, Elmer L. and Richard L. *Bedside Diagnostic Examination*. New York: Macmillan, 1976.

DeMets, David L. *et al.* "A Case Report of Data Monitoring Experience: The Nocturnal Oxygen Therapy Trial." *Controlled Clinical Trials* 3 (1982), 113-124.

Dubos, Rene. *Reason Awake: Science for Man*. New York: Columbia University Press, 1970.

Dupont, William D. "Randomized vs. Historial Clinical Trials." *A.J.Epidemiology* 122:6 (1985), 940-946.

Emanuel, Elliott. "The Art of Medicine. Part III. The Evolution of the Artist." *Canadian Med. Assoc. J.* 119 (November 18, 1978), 1234-1235.

Evans, Mary *et al.* "Trials on Trial: A Review of Trials of Antibiotic Prophylaxis." *Archives of Surgery* 119 (January, 1984), 109-113.

Faber, Knud. "Nosography in Modern Internal Medicine." *Annals of Medical History* IV:I (Spring, 1922), 1-63.

Feinstein, Alvan R. *Clinical Biostatistics*. St. Louis: Mosby, 1977.

_____ ."Clinical Biostatistics IX. How Do We Measure 'Safety' and 'Efficacy?'" *Clin. Pharm. and Ther.* VII (1971), 544-558.

_____ ."Clinical Biostatistics XLVII. Scientific Standards vs. Statistical Associations and Biologic Logic in the Analysis of Causation." *Clin. Pharm. and Ther.* 25:4 (April, 1979), 481-492.

_____."Clinical Epidemiology III. The Clinical Design of Statistics in Therapy." *Annals of Internal Medicine* 69 (1968), 1287-1312.

_____.*Clinical Judgment.* Huntington, N.Y.: Krieger, 1967.

Fisher, Bernard. "Winds of Change in Clinical Trials — from Daniel to Charlie Brown." *Controlled Clinical Trials* 4 (1983), 65-73.

Fletcher, A.E., Hunt, B.M., and Bulpitt, C.J. "Evaluation of Quality of Life in Clinical Trials of Cardiovascular Disease." *J. Chronic Disease* 40:6 (1987), 557-566.

Fletcher, C.M. "The Clinical Diagnosis of Pulmonary Emphysema — an Experimental Study." *Proc. Royal Soc. Med.* 45 (1952), 577.

Fletcher, R.H. and S.W. "Clinical Research in General Medical Journals." *New England J. Med.* 301:4 (July 26, 1979), 180-183.

Fligor, L.W. "The Placebo Effect." *Journal of the AMA* 234:8 (Nov. 24, 1975), 808.

Fredrickson, D.S. "The Field Trial: Some Thoughts on the Indispensable Ordeal." *New York Acad. Med. Bull.* 44:8 (1968), 985-993.

_____."Welcoming Remarks," *Clinical Pharm. and Ther.* 25:5 (May, 1979), Part 2, 630-631.

Friedman, Howard S. "Randomized Clinical Trials and Common Sense." *A. J. Med.* 81 (December, 1986), 1047.

Friedman, L., Wenger, N.K., and Knatterud, G.L. "Impact of the Coronary Drug Project Findings on Clinical Practice." *Controlled Clinical Trials* 4 (1983), 513-522.

Friedman, Paul J. "Correcting the Literature Following Fraudulent Publication." *Journal of the AMA* 263:10 (March 9, 1990), 1416-1419.

Gifford, R.H. and A. Feinstein. "A Critique of Methodology in Studies of Anticoagulent Therapy for Acute Myocardial Infarction." *New England J. Med.* 280 (1969), 351-357.

Goldman, Anne I. *et al.* "Can Dropout and Other Noncompliance Be Minimized in a Clinical Trial?" *Controlled Clinical Trials* 3 (1982), 75-89.

Goodman, A.G. and L.S. and Gilman, A. *The Pharmacological Basis of Therapeutics.* Sixth Edition. New York: Macmillan, 1980.

Gordis, Leon. "Assuring the Quality of Questionnaire Data in Epidemiologic Research." *A.J.Epidemiology* 109:1 (1979), 21-24.

Gordon, R.S. "Clinical Trials." *New England J. Med.* 298:7 (February 16, 1978).

Green, Sylvan B. "Patient Heterogeneity and the Need for Randomized Clinical Trials." *Controlled Clinical Trials* 3 (1982), 189-198.

Grizzle, James E. "A Note on Stratifying Versus Complete Random Assignment in Clinical Trials." *Controlled Clinical Trials* 3 (1982), 365-368.

H.D.R.,Jr. "'Delayed' Iatrogenic Diseases." *Southern M.J.* 67:11 (November, 1974), 1271-1274.

Harris, E.L. and J.D.Fitzgerald. *The Principles and Practice of Clinical Trials. Based on a Symposium Organized by the Association of Medical Advisers in the Pharmaceutical Industry.* Edinburgh and London: E. and S. Livingstone, 1970.

Harvey, A. McGhehee *et al. Principles and Practice of Medicine.* 19th Edition. New York: Appleton-Century-Crofts, 1976.

Herbst, Arthur I., Howard Ulfelder, and David C. Poskanzer. "Adenocarcinoma of the Vagina: Association of Maternal Stilbestrol Therapy with Tumor Appearance in Young Women." *New England J. Med.* 284:16 (1971), 878-881.

Herfindal, E.T. and J.L. Hirschman, eds. *Clinical Pharmacology and Therapeutics.* Baltimore: Williams and Wilkins, 1975.

Herrick, A.D. and McKeen Cattell. *Clinical Testing of New Drugs.* New York: Revere Publishing Co., 1965.

Hill, Austin Bradford. *Controlled Clinical Trials.* Springfield: Thomas, 1960.

_____."Reflections on the Controlled Clinical Trial." *Annals of the Rheumatic Diseases* 25 (1966), 107-113.

Hoffer, Abram. "A Theoretical Examination of Double-Blind Design." *Canadian Med. Assoc. J.* 97 (July 15, 1967), 123-127.

_____ and H. Osmond. "Double-Blind Clinical Trials." *J. Psychiatry* 2 (1960-1961), 221-227.

Hollister, Leo E. *et al.* "Drug Therapy of Depression: Amitriptyline, Perphenazine, and Their Combination in Different Syndromes." *Arch. Gen. Psych.* 17 (1967), 486-493.

Horwitz, Ralph I. "The Experimental Paradigm and Observational Studies of Cause-Effect Relationships in Clinical Medicine." *J. Chron. Dis.* 40:1 (1987), 91-99.

Houston, Robert G. *Repression and Reform in the Evaluation of Alternative Cancer Therapies.* Washington, D.C.: Project Cure, 1987, 1989.

Hutchinson, T.A. *et al.* "Scientific Problems in Clinical Scales, as Demonstrated by the Karnofsky Index of Performance Status." *J. Chron. Dis.* 32 (1979), 661-666.

Institute for Alternative Futures. "Foresight Seminar Summmary: The Cost of Developing Medicines" (December 11, 1989). (unpublished)

Johnson, F. Neil and Susan, eds. *Clinical Trials.* Oxford: Blackwell, 1977.

Jones, Hardin B. "Demographic Considerations of the Cancer Problem." *Trans. New York Acad. Sci.* (February, 1956), 298-333.

Kabat, Elvin A. *Structural Concepts in Immunology and Immunochemistry.* New York: Holt, Rinehart, and Wilson, 1976.

Kapit, Richard M. "Schizophrenia and Tardive Dyskenesia: Is Schizophrenia Also a 'Denervation Hypersensitivity'?" *Medical Hypotheses* III:5 (September-October, 1977), 207-210.

Lasagna, Louis. *Controversies in Therapeutics.* Philadelphia: W.B.Saunders, 1980.

_____ ."Thalidomide—A New Nonbarbiturate Sleep-Inducing Drug." *J. Chron. Dis.* 11:6 (June, 1960), 627-631.

Levine, Robert J. "The Apparent Incompatibility Between Informed Consent and Placebo-Controlled Trials." *Clin.Pharm. and Ther.* 42:3 (September, 1987), 247-249.

Linder, Maria C. "Biochemical Bases for Diversity and Individuality in Human Metabolism: An Overview." In: Karl Schaefer, ed., *New Image of Man in Medicine, Volume II: Basis of an Individual Psychology*. Mount Kisco: Futura Publishing Company, 1979.

Lisook, Alan B. "FDA Investigation of Clinical Studies: Policy and Procedure." Presented at Third Annual European Symposium: Good Clinical Practice in Europe, Copenhagen, Denmark, March 3, 1989. (unpublished)

Mackillop, W.J. and Johnston, P.A. "Controlled Clinical Trials: An Ethical Imperative?" *J. Chron. Dis.* 40:4 (1987), 363.

_____ ."Ethical Problems in Clinical Research: The Need for Empirical Studies of the Clinical Trials Process." *J. Chron. Dis.* 39:3 (1986), 177-188.

McPeek, Bucknam. "Inference, Generalizability, and a Major Change in Anesthetic Practice." *J. Anesthesiology* 66:6 (June, 1987), 723-724.

Maxwell, C. "The Significance of Significance." *Clinical Trials* 5 (1968), 1015-1020.

Medical Research Council. "Streptomycin Treatment of Pulmonary Tuberculosis." *British M.J.* 2 (1948), 769-782.

Meier, Paul. "Stratification in the Design of a Clinical Trial." *Controlled Clinical Trials* I (1980), 355-361.

Meinert, Curtis L. "Toward More Definitive Clinical Trials." *Controlled Clinical Trials* I (1980), 249-261.

Meyer, J.L. "Some Instrument-Induced Errors in the Electrocardiogram." *Journal of the AMA* 201 (1967), 351-356.

Miller, S. T. and Clifton Parry. "New Lessons Favoring Physicians' Support of Clinical Trials." *A.J.Medicine* 77 (September, 1984), 533-536.

Modell, Walter. "The Sensitivity and Validity of Drug Evaluations in Man." *Clinical Pharm. and Ther.* I (1960), 769-776.

Mondzac, A.M. "Throat-Culture Processing in the Office — A Warning." *Journal of the AMA* 200 (1967), 1132.

Moscucci, Mauro *et al.* "Blinding, Unblinding, and the Placebo Effect: An Analysis of Patients' Guesses of Treatment Assignment in a Double-Blind Clinical Trial." *Clin. Pharm. and Ther.* 41:3 (March, 1987), 259-265.

Moser, Marvin. "Treating Hypertension: A Review of Clinical Trials." *A. J. Med.* 81: Supplement 6C. (December 31, 1986), 25-37.

Moss, Ralph. *The Cancer Industry: Unravelling the Politics.* New York: Paragon House, 1989.

National Analysts. *A Study of Health Practices and Opinions.* Philadelphia: National Analysts, 1972.

Nodine, J.H. and P.E.Siegler. *Animal and Clinical Pharmacologic Techniques in Drug Evaluation.* Chicago: Year Book Medical Publishers, 1964.

Northrop, F.S.C. *The Logic of the Sciences and the Humanities.* New York: Meridian Books, 1960.

NOVA. "Do Scientists Cheat?" Broadcast October 25, 1988. WGBH Transcripts, Boston, Massachusetts.

Osler, William. *Principles and Practice of Medicine.* Sixth Edition. New York: Appleton, 1906.

Palmer, Roger, ed. *Controversies in Clinical Pharmacology and Drug*

*Development.* New York: Futura, 1972.

Perkins, W.H. *The Cause and Prevention of Disease.* Philadelphia: Lea and Febiger, 1938.

Pfeifer, Mark P. and G. Snodgrass. "The Continued Use of Retracted Invalid Scientific Literature." *Journal of the AMA* 263:10 (March 9, 1990), 1420-1423.

Pharmaceutical Manufacturers' Association. *Annual Survey Report, 1979-1980.* Washington, D. C.: PMA, 1980a.

_____. *Annual Survey Report, 1987-1989.* Washington, D. C. : PMA, 1990.

_____. *Prescription Drug Industry.* Washington, D. C.: PMA, 1980b.

Platt, Robert. "Doctor and Patient." *Lancet* 1963 (ii), 1156-1158.

Relman, Arnold. "The New Medical-Industrial Complex." *New England J.Med.* 303:17 (October 23, 1980), 963-970.

Rennie, Drummond. "Editors and Auditors." *Journal of the AMA* 261:17 (May 5, 1989), 2543-2545.

Ritchie, D.M. *et al.* "Clinical Studies with an Articular Index for the Assessment of Joint Tenderness in Patients with Rheumatoid Arthritis." *Q. J. Med.* NS 37:147 (July, 1968), 393-406.

Roberts, Robin *et al.* "An Empirical Demonstration of Berkson's Bias." *J. Chron. Dis.* 31 (1978), 119-128.

Ropes, Marian W. *et al.* "Proposed Diagnostic Criteria for Rheumatoid Arthritis." *Bulletin on Rheumatic Diseases* VII:4 (December, 1956), 121-124.

Ross, O.B., Jr. "Nitrate Therapy for Angina Pectoris Still Debated

After 100 Years." *Journal of the AMA* 199 (March 6, 1967), 35-36.

Rutstein, David D. *The Coming Revolution in Medicine.* Cambridge: MIT Press, 1967.

Shapiro, Martin F. and Robert P. Charrow. "The Role of Data Audits in Detecting Scientific Misconduct." *Journal of the AMA* 261:17 (May 5, 1989), 2505-2511.

Siegler, Edward E. "Microdiagnosis of Carcinoma in Situ of the Uterine Cervix. A Comparative Study of Pathologists' Diagnoses." *Cancer* 9 (1956), 463-469.

Silverman, Milton and Philip Lee. *Pills, Profits, and Politics.* Berkeley: University of California, 1974.

Sodeman, W.A. and W.A. Sodeman, Jr. *Pathologic Physiology: Mechanisms of Disease.* Fourth Edition. Philadelphia: W.B.Saunders, 1967.

Special Committee on Internal Pollution. "Toward Assessing the Chemical Age." *Journal of the AMA* 234:5 (November 3, 1975), 507-509.

Spence, James. "The Methodology of Clinical Science." *Lancet* (September 25, 1953), 629-632.

Spodick, David H. "The Randomized Controlled Clinical Trial: Scientific and Ethical Bases." *A.J.Medicine* 73 (September, 1982), 420-425.

Steel, Knight *et al.* "Iatrogenic Illness on a General Medical Service at a University Hospital." *New England J.Med.* 304:11 (March 12, 1981), 638-642.

Stone, George B. "The New Product Challenge." *A.J. Pharmacy* 131 (1959), 327-336.

Strauss, Anselm L. *Chronic Disease and the Quality of Life.* St. Louis:

Mosby, 1975.

Talalay, Paul, ed. *Drugs in Our Society*. Baltimore: Johns Hopkins, 1964.

Tannock, Ian and Kevin Murphy. "Reflections on Medical Oncology: An Appeal for Better Clinical Trials and Improved Reporting of Their Results." *J. Clinical Oncology* 1:1 (January, 1983), 66-70.

Taylor, Kathryn M. *et al.* "Physicians' Reasons for Not Entering Eligible Patients in a Randomized Clinical Trial of Surgery for Breast Cancer." *New England J.Med.* 311:21 (May 24, 1984), 1363-1367.

Thomas, Lewis. "Guessing and Knowing: Reflections on the Science and Technology of Medicine." *Saturday Review* (December 23, 1972), 52-57.

Thomson, Mary Ellen and M.S.Kramer. "Methodologic Standards for Controlled Clinical Trials of Early Contact and Maternal-Infant Behavior." *Pediatrics* 73:3 (March, 1984), 294-299.

Tyson, Jon E. "Therapeutic Studies in Perinatal Medicine." *Obstetrics and Gynecology* 64:2 (August, 1984), 300-301.

_____ .*et al.* "An Evaluation of the Quality of Therapeutic Studies in Perinatal Medicine." *Obstetrics and Gynecology* 62:1 (July, 1983), 99-102.

U.S. Congress. Office of Technology Assessment. *Assessing the Efficacy and Safety of Medical Technologies*. Washington, D.C.: OTA, 1978.

_____ .*Background Paper: The Impact of Randomized Clinical Trials on Health Policy and Medical Practice*. Washington, D.C.: OTA, 1983.

United States Department of Health, Education, and Welfare.

Public Health Service. *International Classification of Diseases*. Eighth Revision. Washington, D.C.: GPO, 1976.

United States Department of Health and Human Services, Public Health Service. *Health United States, 1988*. Washington, D.C., 1989.

United States Senate. Committee on Labor and Public Welfare. Subcommittee on Health. *Examination of the Pharmaceutical Industry, 1973-1974*. Part 5 (May 20, 1974).

_____ .Select Committee on Small Business. Subcommittee on Monopoly. *Competitive Problems in the Drug Industry*. Part 11 (February-March, 1969).

Vandenbroucke, Jan P. "A Short Note on the History of the Randomized Controlled Trial." *J. Chron. Dis.* 40:10 (1987), 985-987.

Vickers, Geoffrey. "Medicine, Psychiatry, and General Practice." *Lancet* (May 15, 1965), 1021-1027.

Vonder Haar, T.A. and Mark Miller. "Warning: Your Prescription May be Dangerous To Your Health." *New York* (May 16, 1977), 46-57.

Wade, Nicholas. "Physicians Who Falsify Data." *Science* 180 (June 8, 1973), 1038.

Weiss, W. and J.M. Dambrosio. "Common Problems in Designing Therapeutic Trials in Multiple Sclerosis." *Archives of Neurology* 40 (October 21, 1983), 678-680.

Whittlesey, Marietta. "The Runaway Use of Antibiotics." *The New York Times Magazine*, May 6, 1979, 122-127.

Williams, Roger. "Normal Young Men." *Persp. Biol. and Med.* I (1957-1958), 97-104.

Wing, J. and J. Nixon. "Discriminating Symptoms in Schizophrenia." *Arch. Gen. Psychiatry* 26 (July, 1975), 853-859.

Witts, L.J. *Medical Surveys and Clinical Trials.* London: Oxford University Press, 1964.

Yeager, Mark P. *et al.,* "Epidural Anesthesia and Analgesia in High-Risk Surgical Patients." *J. Anesthesiology* 66 (1987), 729-736.

Yerushalmy, J. *et al.* "An Evaluation of the Role of Serial Chest Roentgenograms in Estimating the Progress of Disease in Patients with Pulmonary Tuberculosis." *American Review of Tuberculosis* 64 (1951), 225-228.

_____ ."The Role of Dual Reading in Mass Radiography." *American Review of Tuberculosis* 61 (1950), 443-448.

# ABOUT THE AUTHOR

Harris L. Coulter, born in Baltimore in 1932, was a student of politics and economics at Yale and has the Ph.D. in political science from Columbia (1969).

He was preparing for a career in government and diplomacy when, at the age of 28, he became interested in the history of medicine.

He decided to devote himself exclusively to this discipline and, since 1973, has published ten books and several dozen articles on medical history, homoeopathic medicine, vaccination problems, medical education, and, now, the controlled clinical trial.

His major effort, *Divided Legacy: A History of the Schism in Medical Thought*, analyzes medical philosophy from its origins in the writings of Hippocrates to the present day. Planned as a four-volume work, three volumes have already been published, bringing the account up to 1900. He is presently doing the research for Volume IV, which will cover the period, 1900-1990.

Otherwise Dr. Coulter works as an interpreter and translator in the Russian and French languages. He has been a simultaneous interpreter at the United Nations and the U.S. Department of State and has interpreted, in particular, for such well-known Russian political and cultural figures as Alexander Solzhenitsyn, Andrei Sakharov, and Boris Yeltsin.

His wife, Catherine Coulter, is a well-known authority on homoeopathic medicine. They have four children.

## Other Books Available From
## the Center for Empirical Medicine

Coulter, Catherine R. *Portraits of Homoeopathic Medicines: Psychophysical Analyses of Selected Constitutional Types. Volume I.* North Atlantic Books, Wehawken Book Company, Homoeopathic Educational Services, 1986. $25.00. ISBN 0-938190-61-X.

Coulter, Catherine R. *Portraits of Homoeopathic Medicines. Volume II.* North Atlantic Books, Wehawken Book Company, Homoeopathic Educational Services, 1988. $25.00. ISBN 0-938190-61-X.

Coulter, Catherine R. *Portrait of Indifference* (supplement to *Portraits, Volume II*). North Atlantic Books, Wehawken Book Company, Homoeopathic Educational Services, 1989. $6.95. ISBN 1-55643-077-9.

Coulter, Harris L. *Divided Legacy: A History of the Schism in Medical Thought. Volume I. The Patterns Emerge: Hippocrates to Paracelsus.* Wehawken Book Company, 1975. ISBN 0-916386-01-5. *Volume II. The Origins of Modern Western Medicine: J.B. Van Helmont to Claude Bernard.* Wehawken Book Company, North Atlantic Books, 1988. ISBN 1-55643-035-3. *Volume III. The Conflict Between Homoeopathy and the American Medical Association.* Second Edition. North Atlantic Books, 1982. ISBN 0-938190-57-1. $35.00/volume, $105.00/set. Volume III is also available in paperback at $15.00. ISBN 0-913028-96-7.

Coulter, Harris L. *Homoeopathic Medicine.* Formur, Inc., 1975. $1.65. ISBN 0-89378-072-3.

Coulter, Harris L. *Homoeopathic Science and Modern Medicine: the Physics of Healing with Microdoses.* North Atlantic Books and Homoeopathic Educational Services, 1981. $9.95. ISBN 0-913028-84-3.

Coulter, Harris L. *AIDS and Syphilis: the Hidden Link.* North Atlantic Books, Wehawken Book Co., 1987. $8.95. ISBN 1-55643-021-3. Also available in hardback at $19.95.

Coulter, Harris L. *Vaccination, Social Violence, and Criminality: the Medical Assault on the American Brain.* North Atlantic Books, Wehawken Book Company, 1990. $15.00. ISBN 1-55643-0841-1. Also available in hardback at $25.00.

Coulter, Harris L. and Barbara Loe Fisher. *DPT: A Shot in the Dark.* Second Edition. Avery Publishing Group. (forthcoming, Spring, 1991)

Please enclose payment with order, adding 10% (15% on foreign orders) for postage.

Center For Empirical Medicine
4221 45th Street NW
Washington, DC 20016
(202) 362-3185
(202) 364-0898

# ABOUT PROJECT CURE

Founded as a grass roots political movement by cancer patients in 1979, Project Cure is today one of the largest and most effective health lobbying organizations in America. Its mission is to furnish Americans with the truth so they can make the right choices about treatment for cancer and other life threatening diseases. It works to expose conspiracy and fraud within the medical establishment and to bring more public attention to exciting frontiers in alternative cancer therapy.

Project Cure does not specifically advocate any one method of treatment. Instead, it believes Americans must be free to choose the treatment they prefer after considering *all* of the available options, both within the United States and abroad.

Project Cure was instrumental in lobbying Congress to investigate alternative cancer treatments currently in use here and in foreign countries. The Congressional Office of Technology Assessment's lengthy report, issued in 1990, confirmed that many therapies that are outside mainstream medicine may be effective and should be investigated further. Armed with these findings, Project Cure is now lobbying Congress and the National Cancer Institute to initiate research into the most promising alternative treatments and determine, once and for all, whether our nation's War on Cancer is, in fact, misdirected and off course. We are supported solely by contributions from those who are interested in this vital question.

Project Cure
1101 Connecticut Ave. NW
Suite 403
Washington, DC 20036